EMOTIONAL
INTELLIGENCE
IN NURSING

Estelle Codier, PhD, MSN, RN, published one of the first nursing research studies demonstrating the relationship between emotional intelligence and clinical performance in nursing. Over 15 years, her further research examined the relationship between EI and nurse retention, gender, generational differences, culture, and educational outcomes. She is the author of over three dozen peer-reviewed articles, book chapters, and conference proceedings and has presented her research at conferences across the globe. Her interest in innovative methods for teaching EI abilities led her to write a textbook on teaching in virtual space, which includes a chapter on teaching EI ability in a virtual environment.

Retired as an associate professor from the University of Hawaii, Manoa, Dr. Codier's current interest is in developing EI capabilities of nurses, particularly in their impact on resiliency, wellness, and salutogenic practices. Dr. Codier resides in the Pacific Northwest with her husband.

EMOTIONAL INTELLIGENCE IN NURSING

ESSENTIALS FOR LEADERSHIP AND PRACTICE IMPROVEMENT

Estelle Codier, PhD, MSN, RN

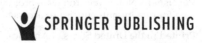 SPRINGER PUBLISHING

Springer Publishing Company, LLC
11 West 42nd Street, New York, NY 10036
www.springerpub.com
connect.springerpub.com/

Acquisitions Editor: Rachel X. Landes
Compositor: Amnet Systems

ISBN: 978-0-8261-7453-6
ebook ISBN: 978-0-8261-7454-3
DOI: 10.1891/9780826174543

20 21 22 23 / 5 4 3 2 1

The author and the publisher of this Work have made every effort to use sources believed to be reliable to provide information that is accurate and compatible with the standards generally accepted at the time of publication. The author and publisher shall not be liable for any special, consequential, or exemplary damages resulting, in whole or in part, from the readers' use of, or reliance on, the information contained in this book. The publisher has no responsibility for the persistence or accuracy of URLs for external or third-party Internet websites referred to in this publication and does not guarantee that any content on such websites is, or will remain, accurate or appropriate.

Library of Congress Cataloging-in-Publication Data

Names: Codier, Estelle, author.
Title: Emotional intelligence in nursing : essentials for leadership and
   practice improvement / Estelle Codier.
Description: New York, NY : Springer Publishing Company, LLC, [2021] |
   Includes bibliographical references and index. |
Identifiers: LCCN 2020037549 (print) | LCCN 2020037550 (ebook) | ISBN
   9780826174536 (paperback) | ISBN 9780826174543 (ebook)
Subjects: MESH: Nursing Care—psychology | Emotional Intelligence |
   Leadership | Clinical Competence | Nurse-Patient Relations
Classification: LCC RT41 (print) | LCC RT41 (ebook) | NLM WY 87 | DDC
   610.73—dc23
LC record available at https://lccn.loc.gov/2020037549
LC ebook record available at https://lccn.loc.gov/2020037550

Contact sales@springerpub.com to receive discount rates on bulk purchases.

Printed in the United States of America.

In 2020, millions of nurses worldwide went to work every day knowing they were risking their lives to care for patients with COVID-19. They were afraid but courageously chose to care anyway. To these nurses, to those who became ill as a result, and to those who died, the world owes an incalculable debt.

This book is dedicated to them.

CONTENTS

PROLOGUE:
MESSAGE IN A BOTTLE

It was one of those times at the bedside that I will never forget. The story haunted me like the koan a spiritual master gives a student to ponder endlessly. The details were clear, but the message was impenetrable. I carried the story in my mental pocket, rubbing it like a touchstone, as I struggled to articulate its true meaning for years.

One of my clinical students had called me to the bedside of a patient, admitted for end-stage renal disease, who was refusing care. He was refusing breakfast, a bath, and medications. However, the patient was not refusing to have a student care for him, which, given the other refusals, I would have expected. He was not refusing contact.

People with end-stage renal disease, which can ravage both length and quality of life, wrestle with these issues. They are often labeled as difficult and often are. The student was one of my best—he had done everything he could. I went to the bedside rehearsing the "Sometimes there isn't a lot you can do for these patients" talk I anticipated later having with the student.

I entered the room and greeted the patient, who mostly ignored me. I greeted the student hovering on the other side of the bed. I sat in a chair, threw my arm over the siderail, and nonchalantly leaned forward. The patient was too far down in the bed, looking emotionally sour and physically uncomfortable. It was hard to resist the temptation to swoop in and adjust his body and bed to approximate my notion of comfort. Instead, I introduced myself and reached over casually to adjust his cooked nasal canula, which was pressing against his nostril at an angle. "That can't be comfortable." I said. I nodded to the breakfast tray, untouched on the table in front of him. "Are you sure I can't tempt you with some breakfast?"

The patient shook his head.

I replied, "Cold eggs. I can't imagine why not."

The patient grunted in response, a hint of amusement in his expression at my attempt at sarcasm.

I prattled on about getting out of bed and later about the importance of preventing pneumonia. No response. I was role modeling futility.

But then I started, "So, before all this ..." waving my hand around his body, the room, "What did you do for work?"

The patient paused, taken aback. He shifted in bed slightly, adjusting himself. He made eye contact. He cleared his throat. "I was a 911 call operator."

Now, so many years later, I can still hear his voice: *"I was a 911 call operator."*

A tingle spread across my skin. I held his gaze for a moment and shook my head. I turned away from him, catching the student's eye instead. "Do you have any idea what that means?"

The student, a bit confused, said, "Well, not really."

I told the student about 911 call operators, about how the 911 operator stays on the phone with the person in trouble after calling the ambulance, fireman, or police, about how the voice of the 911 operator holds onto them, stays with them, amid whatever horribleness the person is experiencing, until help arrives. When assistance comes, the operator signs off, answers the next call, and holds on, again, to the next person. They do this over, and over, and over again, all day, every workday. I talked about the stress, the burnout rate, and the cost of working in that kind of intensity day after day. I talked about how incredibly important experienced 911 operators are.

In the middle of this, while I was "ignoring" the patient and focusing on my lecture to the student, I saw the change out of the corner of my eye. The patient shifted in bed. His posture straightened. He sat up taller. When I turned back to him, the eyes that met mine were clear and calm.

I ended the mini-lecture for my student and asked the patient, "So, let me ask you this: I have helped train medic response units forever ... how the heck did you do it for all those years?"

The patient shrugged, not meeting my eyes. "You just do it."

I told him I was interested in talking with him more later. "How about we warm up these eggs for you?"

The man nodded as the student reached for the tray.

When I rose to leave, I said over my shoulder, "If you can deal with being a 911 operator, you can deal with this, you know that, right?"

The patient simply reached for his newspaper and nodded again.

In the hall, the student reached for my arm and said, "How did you know that was the question to ask?"

Because I didn't have a clue how I had known, I instead asked the student what he saw happen.

He said, "Because of your question, he remembered who he was."

I don't know what happened next to the patient. Maybe he continued to refuse care. Maybe he *did* remember who he was as well as his ability to adapt and cope. Maybe he remembered his dignity and importance. Maybe he didn't.

But how *did* I know that was the question to ask? I had no idea. It is a huge part of nursing, that *thing* we do. It's hunch, intuition, magic, a mystery, a miracle. While maturing as a professional, I gave this phenomenan many names. I understood finally it was not unique to nursing. Helping a person in trouble tap into their own capabilities is an important first step to supporting them as they grapple with challenges, physical or emotional. But still, how had I known to ask that one question?

The various answers I came up with, (Intuition! Precognitive awareness! Advanced assessment capabilities!) were never enough. I always believed in that *thing*, not unique to nursing but fundamental to excellent nursing practice, at the bedside, in teams, in education, and in nursing leadership. That *thing* not only defined an exceptional part of being a nurse, it also helped differentiate between outstanding nurses and nurses going through the motions. I wanted to know what that thing was. I wanted to understand it. I wanted to know its name.

I ended up in a PhD program by accident. While I was away on leave for a family emergency, my supervisor assigned me to a joint appointment between the hospital, where I was a critical nurse educator, and the local university nursing school. "Usually, we donate money to the university," he explained. "This time, we want to donate you." I was to be part-time nurse educator, part-time university faculty. I was not pleased. However, it did come with free PhD tuition. Research, after all, is just a systematic way of answering questions, and goodness knows, I had questions. I wasn't sure how to pick a PhD research topic, so my PhD advisor asked if I had any burning questions about nursing. I felt that 911 operator touchstone story heavy in the pocket of my mind. Yes, I did.

My studies led me to *gnosis*, the wonderful Greek word for "knowledge learned from living, not reading or studying." How do nurses develop nursing gnosis? Nurses talk a lot about assessment, problem-solving, and critical thinking, but before all that, how do we "gnose"? How do nurses synthesize what they learn from reading and study with what they learned from living, from patients every working day? Some heavy philosophy reading guided me through "thinking about thinking," and later to the field of intelligence theory. One day, among the library stacks, I found *the* book. It was titled *Emotional Intelligence*.

I took the book home. I did not read it for almost 3 months, staring at the title every day and wondering. In that time, the architecture of my understanding about what nursing is was undone, and, piece by piece, rebuilt. What if emotional intelligence was what I had been trying to name, all those years, that thing that had defied a name? What if nursing excellence is not about personality, values, grade point average, or even professionalism? What if what nurses often call intuition is a deep, often precognitive form of pattern recognition, neither magic nor miracle, but rather very specific and measurable intelligence? What if it could be taught, learned, developed? What would this mean for nursing, both conceptually and practically? What could it mean for nursing recruitment, education, and practice?

The die was cast. My PhD work focused on the nascent field of emotional intelligence (EI) in nursing. My simple study, one of the earliest on nurse performance and EI, was the first to provide evidence for the relationship between EI ability and clinical performance. I continued my research, wrote many articles, and made dozens of presentations to nurses across the globe. Now, it is time to take stock. What do we know so far? What could it mean? What could be ahead?

This book was undertaken to:

1. Provide a conceptual and historical description of EI as a concept and its application to nursing practice;
2. In a very specific and granular manner, illustrate the use of EI abilities across various aspects of nursing practice (See chapter titles for these aspects);
3. Describe the current evolution of the body of nurse EI research, including a summary of both the existing evidence and opportunities for future research; and
4. Offer ideas about how to develop EI abilities.

Chapters 1 and 2 constitute the foundation for this work. In Chapter 1, a history of the evolution of EI as a concept is presented alongside the philosophical and social context. The main models of EI are introduced, with a brief discussion of instrumentation and issues related to the models. Chapter 2 reviews the physiological basis of emotions and emotional responses, as well as an introduction to the "anatomy" of emotions, that is, a structure for understanding them. The bulk of the remaining chapters focus on an aspect of nursing practice and apply the foundation material specifically through stories from nursing practice to illustrate the use (and sometimes failure to use!) EI abilities.

The chapters may be used individually or collectively. To that end, every chapter has a similar structure: each begins by restating the operational definitions of EI on which the chapter material is based. The goals of the chapter are reviewed briefly. In the main body of each chapter, the four basic EI abilities are applied to chapter topics, including both clinical and conceptual content. Often, integration with related existing theory is presented. Stories and reflection on the stories are used to specifically illustrate the concepts presented. Each chapter ends with general references to relevant research findings, which are detailed with specific references in Chapter 15 and a sample exercise to develop EI ability.

The book concludes with two summary chapters. Chapter 15 presents a descriptive summary of the first 20 years of nursing EI research. In the final chapter, "Epilogue," the role of EI in the future of nursing after the COVID-19 pandemic is presented.

To you the reader, for your excellence, for your thriving, this book is offered.

Estelle Codier, PhD, MSN, RN
Overlooking Discovery Bay,
Port Townsend, Washington,
Spring, 2021

ACKNOWLEDGMENTS

In gratitude

Nursing has been a profession that "ate its young." As young kids growing up in the country, we used to stand on each other's shoulders. We did it to climb over obstacles or to see far ahead. Nursing is more like that now, and it has been like that for me. Each of the following wonderful people, each in their own way and usually "just in time," patted their shoulder and said to me, "come on up." Without their partnership, help, and encouragement, this work would not have been possible:

Dr. "Bee" Kooker
Dr. Ruey Ryburn
Dr. Vickie Niederhauser
Dr. Carolyn Constantin
Dr. Kristin Akerjordet, Norway
Dr. Zaid Al Hamdan, Jordan
Art Gladstone, RN, MSN
Cindy Kamikawa, RN, MSN
David Codier, RN, BSN

And to my husband, Buddy Summers, my partner in everything.

1

Introduction to Emotional Intelligence

INTRODUCTION

This chapter introduces emotional intelligence (EI), providing a foundation for the remaining text chapters. It includes:

1. A review of the evolution of EI and its place within intelligence theory.
2. The societal context that gave rise to its evolution.
3. A review of several EI models, with a discussion of their salient differences.
4. A brief summary of early EI research.
5. The case for use of the ability EI model in nursing.

A BRIEF HISTORY OF EMOTIONAL INTELLIGENCE

In the early 1990s, two cognitive psychologists, Doctors John D. Mayer and Peter Salovey, began to study the relationship between cognition and emotional functioning. Mayer and Salovey identified a subgroup of individuals different from their other study participants. These people did not separate cognition and emotions, but instead wove the two together, thinking and feeling in unison. Their emotions informed cognition and cognition informed their emotions. The group was different in other ways. At work, they were high performers, and other measures of life success were also higher. Doctors Mayer and Salovey named this difference "emotional intelligence" (EI) (Salovey & Mayer, 1990).

They defined EI as the "ability to recognize the meanings of emotions .... and to reason and problem-solve on the basis of them" (Mayer et al., 1999, p. 267). Their EI model, and the instruments developed to measure it (first the MEIS and later the MSCEIT) were revised, adapted, and

1

improved over more than a decade. Other researchers developed other EI models, but it is the Mayer and Salovey's ability model that is used as the foundation for this text. In this model, EI is operationally defined with the following abilities: (1) accurate identification of emotions in self and others, (2) understanding emotions, (3) using emotions to reason (integrating thinking and feeling), and (4) managing emotions (Mayer et al., 1999). (*Note: For the purposes of this text, skills 2 and 3 are reversed from the published Mayer et al. order. This is done to better align the four abilities with the nursing process illustrated throughout this chapter.)

Each of these abilities is supported by a wide range of emotional, cognitive, and emotional abilities. For example, identifying an emotion accurately depends on skills such as the ability to correctly read and interpret facial expressions, nonverbal communication, body language, and vocal inflections. Understanding emotions involves skills as varied as appreciation of the antecedents, meanings, and consequences of particular emotions, and interpretation of cultural nuance. Using emotions to reason may include the ability to generate emotions to shift cognitive perspective or to better understand another person's experience. Managing emotions has many supporting skills, such as the ability to promote emotions that are helpful and to disengage from those that are not (Mayer et al., 2016).

Mayer and Salovey's research was published in psychology articles in professional journals. It was first presented to the general public in a book by Daniel Goleman, whose book drew heavily on their research. Goleman, psychologist by training and a journalist by trade, was interested in the role of emotional management in organizations. He wrote a book tentatively titled *Emotional Competency*. His publisher insisted the book was great, but the title was not! Goleman received Mayer and Salovey's permission to title his book *Emotional Intelligence*. The book targeted a general, not professional, audience and sold widely in the United States and worldwide. It was eventually translated into 30 languages and sold over 5 million copies. This was an unprecedented success for what was essentially a book on workplace psychosocial skills. Those two words, "emotional intelligence" hit a nerve.

Goleman's book represented a tipping point. Ideas about not only intelligence, but about emotions and their role in the workplace, had begun to change. These two words, *emotional intelligence,* stirred the public imagination. Like small pebbles starting an avalanche, those two words created a cascade of change in thinking about intelligence and emotions.

These exciting changes reflected a developing consensus that emotions play a significant role in intelligence. The term Mayer and Salovey had coined, "emotional intelligence" offered language to describe this. A new concept was born, but there was no agreement about its definition or how to measure it. Researchers like doctors Mayer and Salovey were interested in EI as an emotional cognitive ability. Others, like Reuven

Bar-On, who worked in community health, and Daniel Goleman, who focused on organizations, conceptualized EI as a combination of ability and other factors such as personality and social function (Bar-On, 2006; Goleman, 1995). These early proponents of EI disagreed on the definition, operational characteristics, and means to measure EI.

DEFINING EMOTIONAL INTELLIGENCE

In this text, Mayer and Salovey's ability EI model is used. EI is defined as an "ability to recognize the meanings of emotions ... and to reason and problem-solve on the basis of them" (Mayer et al., 1999, p. 267).

This definition is operationalized with the following skills:

1. accurate identification of emotions in self and others,
2. understanding emotions,
3. using emotions to reason (integrating thinking and feeling), and
4. managing emotions (Mayer et al., 1997).

In this text, the second and third abilities are reversed from their usual order as outlined by Mayer (Mayer et al., 1997), as this order aligns better with the nursing processes illustrated throughout this work.

Despite the differences between these EI models, EI has continued to be a subject of research in dozens of professional disciplines. It has also become a household word among the general public, both in the United States and across the globe. How did this concept emerge so quickly? What changes in ideas about intelligence set the stage for this rapid change in ideas about the relationship between emotions and cognition and between thinking and feeling?

THINKING ABOUT THINKING: ASSUMPTIONS ABOUT INTELLIGENCE

Disciplines interested in intelligence, such as education, philosophy, and psychology, among others, have always disagreed about the definition, nature, effects, and characteristics of intelligence. However, particularly in western culture, most definitions share a few fundamental assumptions.

Intelligence Has a Hereditary Foundation

Long before scientists understood the intricacies of genetics, most people believed intelligence was inherited. Smart parents gave birth to smart children. Not-so-smart parents gave birth to less smart children. Intelligence was viewed as a trait, like hair color or body build. Mom and her kids all have red hair and the whole family is smart! As the field of genetics developed, however, no "smart gene" was discovered. Yet this assumption about the primarily genetic foundation for intelligence endures, despite the lack of scientific evidence for it.

The Mind Is Separate From Emotion

If mind and body are separate, then cognition (a function of the mind) and emotion (a function of physiology) are also separate. The philosopher Rene Descartes first articulated this theory. Later known as Cartesian dualism, this distinct dialectic between emotion and intelligence became one of the foundations of western philosophy and an essential tenant of western medicine. Proponents of Cartesian dualism believe objective reality can only be perceived unemotionally. In medicine, terms like "psychosomatic illness" reflect Cartesian dualism. The message to patients with physical illnesses caused by emotional distress was, "it is all in your head" (Bynum et al., 2004).

This mind/body and cognition/emotion separation implies conflict between these functions. Rational thought is assumed to be devoid of emotion. Emotions are regarded as contaminants to reason, or "noise" clouding rational thought. Objective, scientific, rational thinking is assumed to be emotionless, and cognition influenced by emotions is suspect. Measurable, objective data are the only data accepted in scientific research. For example, unmeasurable subjective data, like cultural, relational, or phenomenological data, have not been accepted for PhD research until very recently.

Gender issues complicate this dualism. Historically, women were presumed to be more emotional and less rational than men. Opposers to women's voting rights largely thought women were less capable of rational judgments. Terms like "hysteria" were based on hyster, or the uterus. Men, whose rational nature was presumed, were discouraged from an "irrational" emotional life, contributing to emotional repression, which the American Psychological Association lists in their guidelines for identifying toxic masculinity (APA, 2018). Contemporary philosophers have challenged Cartesian dualism with concepts like the "mindbody," which reflected integration of body and mind (Whpoteat.org, 2020).

Intelligence Does Not Change Over Time

As a fixed trait, housed in the mind, intelligence was regarded as a feature of a person's biological nature, and not changeable. Despite the influences of learning, education, and life experience that would seem to render this assumption preposterous, the fixed trait assumption persists.

Intelligence Can Be Accurately Measured

In many ways the most problematic assumption is that intelligence can be accurately measured and these measurements can reliably predict outcomes in professional achievement, academic standing, and a wide of lifetime success measures performance. Over time, the predictive ability of intelligence testing was never sufficiently validated. Despite this, high stakes decisions, such as academic placement, who will go to college, and which professions an individual has access to, have all been controlled by various forms of intelligence testing. In some countries, admission to professional schools is impossible without certain threshold test scores.

Recent research has provided evidence that the predictive usefulness of these tests is largely overstated. In fact, intelligence tests do not have the predictive value presumed in the past. Within the normal range of intelligence, distinctions between intelligence and standardized testing scores do not predict academic or professional success or who will live satisfying and happy lives. They cannot be reliably used across cultural and sociological groups. The research on this is extensive, contradictory, and conflicting. Consequently, many graduate schools no longer require standardized tests of applicants, and their use for undergraduate admissions has decreased dramatically. Nonetheless, IQ and standardized testing continues to be a multibillion-dollar industry in the United States.

CHANGING ASSUMPTIONS ABOUT INTELLIGENCE, MIND, AND BODY

Slowly, over the last 100 years, ideas about intelligence, cognition, and their relationship with emotions and social relationships began to change. By the late 1800s the emerging field of intelligence research supported this. Long-held assumptions began to be examined for research evidence to support or contradict them. Consider the assumption of intelligence as an inherited trait. Albert Einstein was born to parents of average intelligence. Often, prodigies are born to parents with no skill at all in the field of their child's genius. The inherited trait assumption of intelligence does not explain this. Similarly, a child who struggles with learning, or has a learning deficit, may be born to brilliant parents. Research on "gifted" individuals challenges the inherited intelligence theory. The book *Outliers* presents research on such people, concluding that what these individuals had in common was not, in fact, a "gift," but rather approximately 10,000 hours of practice (Gladwell, 2011).

The inherited trait view not only does not hold up against research findings, but it also doesn't pass a common sense "sniff test." Terms like "book smart" and "street smart" reflect this. Who is more intelligent? A person who can memorize facts for an exam, or a person who can tackle complex problems, think on their feet, and problem solve in the real world? On the basis of 50 years of intelligence research, the view of intelligence as a process of critical thinking, problem-solving, ambiguity tolerance, and continuous learning has gained popularity in the general public and credence among researchers.

Nature Versus Nurture

This shift constellated into the "nature versus nurture" debate. Evidence shows, in addition to familial characteristics, intelligence is affected by environment, motivation, and many social, cultural, and interpersonal factors. "Smart" parents who love learning often create environments for their children that foster creativity, intellectual stimulation, and a family culture of continuous learning. A child can "get" their smarts from their family, but via the family culture, not necessarily the family genes. A child born into poverty may have the opposite experience, including lack of access to foods that support a growing brain. That child "got" their intelligence from the family culture as well.

The "nature versus nurture" debate ended in a tie. Genetics has a role in intelligence, but so does curiosity, a love of learning, nutrition, rich learning environments, and varied social and educational experiences. What did get lost as the "nature versus nurture" debate raged was the assumption that intelligence is primarily an inherited trait. The public backlash to the book *The Bell Curve* (Fraser, 1995), which doubled down on the genetic basis of intelligence, reflected this large-scale public shift in ideas about intelligence. That backlash, coupled with the acclaim Goleman's book received, published shortly after *The Bell Curve*, reflects how pervasive this shift had become.

Social/Emotional Intelligence

In the early 1900s, the social/emotional dimension of intelligence began to make inroads into traditional intelligence theory. Scholars included social/emotional processing in their ideas about functioning intelligently in the world. Robert Thorndike, an early intelligence theorist, described intelligence in three parts: abstract intelligence, practical intelligence, and social intelligence (Thorndike, 1920).

In the 1940s, David Weschler, the founder of today's IQ test, included "non-intellective" factors in his own theory of intelligence. Weschler believed these factors "determined the degree of effectiveness intelligence has when used in daily life" (Haggbloom et al., 2002). These factors were not included in the standardized IQ test used nearly universally to quantify intelligence. Nonetheless, the artificial divide between reason and emotion, rooted in Cartesian dualism and reinforced by cultural sexism and class stereotyping, was breaking down. In 2000, intelligence theorist Robert Sternberg stated that a model of intelligence representing only cognitive factors, excluding social and interpersonal ones, did not fully represent human intelligence (Sternberg et al., 2000).

Multifaceted Intelligence

Since the early 1900s, scholars have struggled with defining the nature of intelligence itself. General intelligence theory described intelligence as a singular phenomenon, a unified subject. Thorndike, and later Howard Gardner, described intelligence as multifaceted (Gardner, 1999). Multifaceted intelligence implies people might express intelligence differently. A "street smart" person may not express much abstract intelligence but could outshine their professor with social or practical intelligence. The idea became fully developed with the 1999 publication of Howard Gardner's book *Multiple Intelligences* (Gardner, 1999).

Multiple Intelligences

Gardner originally posited seven primary kinds of intelligence, later expanded to nine (see Figure 1.1). According to Gardner, people draw on

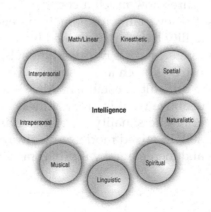

FIGURE 1.1 Multiple intelligences.
Source: Adapted from Gardner, H. (1999). *Intelligence reframed: Multiple intelligences for the 21st century*. Basic Books.

different intelligences. A professional ballroom dancer might primarily express interpersonal, kinesthetic, and musical intelligence. An innovative architect might use spatial, math/linear, and intrapersonal intelligences. Gardener viewed these intelligences as abilities that could be developed and improved over time. He also posited that they also affect the way individuals processes information, learn, and solve problems (Gardner, 1999). Two of the intelligences, interpersonal intelligence (intelligence used in interactions between *people*), and intra personal intelligence (intelligence a person uses in interactions with themself), became the theoretical foundation of what would later be called emotional intelligence.

CRITICAL ISSUES AMONG EI MODELS

As EI evolved as a field of research, various models and definitions were proposed. After 25 years of concept development, the most prevalent models of EI are:

1. EI as an ability, measured by ability testing.
2. EI as an ability, measured by self-report.
3. EI as a mixture of ability and other characteristics.

These models differ in important ways and understanding the critical issues these differences suggest is important.

Instrument Validity

Construct validity measures how much a construct is what it says it is. Is EI a valid thing or is it a new name for something else? The Mayer and Salovey model, being ability based and defined by a few basic abilities, is easy to defend as a discrete concept. EI mixed models, which combine EI abilities with other constructs, such as personality or social ability, make construct validity more difficult to establish. Also, if a test does not measure anything over and above what is already measurable using existing instruments, such as various personality instruments, incremental validity is at issue. For this reason, EI mixed models will always be subject to concerns about construct and incremental validity (Brackett & Mayer, 2003).

EI Instrumentation

Ability instruments, such as the Mayer-Salovey-Caruso Emotional Intelligence Test (MSCEIT), measure emotional abilities. They measure performance of emotional tasks. A test taker is shown a face and asked to identify the emotion expressed. This is vastly different when compared with a self-report instrument, which relies on the test taker's self-evaluation. Self-report findings are only as valid as the test taker's self-assessment is accurate. Such self-assessment is not compared with or validated by any other outside measure. It is well documented in the self-report critique literature that some people habitually rate themselves higher than others, and that some people habitually rate themselves lower. This type of instrument reports self-perception, not actual performance.

A 360-degree instrument relies only on feedback from other people. An EI evaluation at work, for example, could be made up of feedback from an individual's peers, supervisor, and subordinates. This type of testing has some problems. Is a worker's evaluation of their boss ever accurate? Their evaluation may be influenced by power differential issues or a wide range of social/emotional biases. A peer's evaluation could be affected by emotional and social factors such as competition, friendship, and jealousy. A supervisor may have limited opportunity to actually observe their employee working with people so may thus have impressions but not actual data. Instruments that measure performance and 360-degree feedback measure different things (Healthfield, 2019).

The "Apples and Oranges" Problem

As the body of EI research grew rapidly, conclusions from the research evidence became difficult to interpret. Commonly, meta-analyses of EI research included research that utilized dozens of different EI instruments. Findings from research studies examining the same research questions were difficult to compare when they used different definitions of EI and different EI instruments. This "apples and oranges" problem persists in both the general EI research literature and nursing EI research, posing a challenge for meta-analysis and other analytical comparisons of EI research findings.

NURSING AND THE ABILITY MODEL

Across the first 20 years of nursing EI research, a wide range of EI models and instruments were used. This reflected the evolution of EI over those years (Conte, 2005). Some EI instruments are more practical to use than others, as they do not require specialized training or purchase. Others require certification to administer and are available only for purchase. This author recommends the MSCEIT, authored by Mayer, Salovey, and their colleague Caruso, and based on their ability model, this recommendation is based on the following:

Instrumentation Validity and Reliability

At this point in the development of EI instrumentation, the ability instruments, particularly the MSCEIT, v2, have had the most documentation of their validity and reliability. The MSCEIT has undergone instrument testing revision, and its validity and reliability is well-established (Brackett & Mayer, 2003).

Congruence With Nursing Theory

The ability EI model fits well with existing nursing theory. Imogene King's theory, for example, describes emotional abilities as necessary for both therapeutic relationships and effective organizational management (King, 1981).

Congruence With Nursing Process

The ability model, grounded in cognitive and performance elements, meshes well with the nursing process at the core of professional nursing. EI as a way to operationalize emotional problem-solving merges seamlessly with the nursing process.

Operationalizing Caring

The concept of caring is arguably the center of professional nursing, yet it has never been well-explicated or operationalized. The ability EI model and its constituent defining characteristics provide one way to operationalize this concept for nursing.

EI Within a Practice Profession

There is no doubt that personality and social abilities such as empathy and motivation impact the delivery of nursing care. However, both research and clinical use of EI suggest the skills described in the ability model represent distinct functional practice behaviors that explain the effectiveness of nursing interventions. As a practice profession, the ability-based performance EI model could be used as a framework for the evaluation of behaviors required for nursing practice.

STRUCTURE OF THE MSCEIT

Although there are numerous instruments for measuring ability EI, none are as well-established nor as well-tested as the MSCEIT. The MSCEIT instrument measures a total EI score and seven sub-scores, illustrated in Figure 1.2. Total EI comprises two composite scores, Experiential EI and Strategic EI. Experiential EI represents accuracy in perceiving and responding to emotional information. As a composite score, it is based on two subscores, Identification of Emotions and Using Emotions to Reason. The second composite score, Strategic EI, focuses on perceived emotional data. It is made up of two subscores, Understanding Emotions and Managing Emotions. The four EI skills are measured directly and reported as subscores (Identifying, Understanding, Using, and Managing Emotions). They are based on a variety of specific tasks (interpretation of facial expressions, for example; Mayer et al., 2003).

RESEARCHING AND DEVELOPING EI

In the first decade of interdisciplinary EI research, the variety of EI definitions, models, and instruments complicated the comparison of research findings. Despite this, findings from over a hundred research studies across many different disciplines were stunning. Early EI research clearly identified evidence for a correlation between EI and job performance. From salespeople to military personnel, yacht crews, call center workers, and construction workers, higher levels of EI were associated with better performance. Meta-analytic data from EI performance studies provided

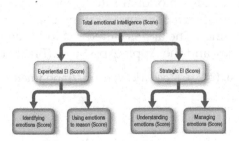

FIGURE 1.2 Ability EI model/MSCEIT score structure.
Source: From Mayer, J. D., Salovey, P., Caruso, D. R., & Sitarenios, G. (2003). Measuring emotional intelligence with the MSCEIT V2. 0. *Emotion, 3*(1), 97–105. https://doi.org/10.1037/1528-3542.3.1.97

clear evidence for this correlation (Cote & Miners, 2006; Joseph & Newman, 2010; Joseph et al., 2015; O'Boyle et al., 2011).

EI was also found to correlate with workplace management abilities and job satisfaction and health. In one meta-analytic review of nearly 20,000 participants, EI was predictive of health outcomes (Martins et al., 2010). Early studies of EI within organizations similarly found associations between EI and effective leadership as well as organizational outcomes such as teamwork, employee and customer satisfaction, employee wellness, job turnover, workplace safety, and even fiscal success (Abraham, 2005; Sánchez-Álvarez et al., 2016; Schutte et al., 2007).

DEVELOPING EI

Three research summaries reviewed a total of 132 EI studies examining the impact of interventions to improve EI. All concluded that many interventions caused lasting EI improvement (Hodzic et al., 2017; Kotsou et al., 2019; Mattingly & Kraiger, 2019). The "apples and oranges" problem pervades these analyses. In one study, over 20 different EI instruments were used across the 46 studies included in the review (Kotsou et al., 2019).

DEVELOPING EMOTIONAL INTELLIGENCE

SAMPLE EMOTIONAL INTELLIGENCE DEVELOPMENT EXERCISE #1: THERE IS EVEN AN APP FOR THIS!

Dr. Mark Brackett, an early collaborator with Mayer, Salovey, and Caruso, founded the first university emotional intelligence laboratory at Yale University. Its current director, Dr. Brackett, has focused recently on social/emotional intelligence in children, developing the RULER EI (Recognize, Understand, Label, Express, Regulate EI) development approach to emotional intelligence . The app he and his colleague Dr. Robin Stern developed can be used as a daily exercise to develop EI abilities. The app is called "Mood Meter" and is available on GooglePlay and the Apple App Store (Brackett, 2020).

Source: Brackett, M. (2020). *Mood Meter*. http://moodmeterapp.com/

REFERENCES

Abraham, R. (2005). Emotional intelligence in the workplace: a review and synthesis. In Schultze, R. & Roberts, R. D. (Eds.), *Emotional intelligence: An international handbook* (p. 255). Hogrefe & Huber Publishers.

American Psychological Association, Boys and Men Guidelines Group. (2018). *APA guidelines for psychological practice with boys and men.* https://www.apa.org /about/policy/boys-men-practice-guidelines.pdf

Bar-On, R. (2006). The Bar-On model of emotional-social intelligence (ESI). *Psicothema, 18,* 13–25.

Brackett, M. A. (2020). *Mood Meter.* http://moodmeterapp.com/

Brackett, M. A., & Mayer, J. D. (2003). Convergent, discriminant, and incremental validity of competing measures of emotional intelligence. *Personality and Social Psychology Bulletin, 29,* 1147–1158. https://doi.org/10.1177/0146167203254596

Bynum, W. F., Shepherd, M., & Porter, R. (2004). *Anatomy of madness* (Vol. 1). Routledge. https://doi.org/10.4324/9781315017099

Conte, J. M. (2005). A review and critique of emotional intelligence measures. *Journal of Organizational Behavior, 26,* 433–440. https://doi.org/10.1002/job.319

Cote, S., & Miners, C. T. H. (2006). Emotional intelligence, cognitive intelligence and job performance. *Administrative Science Quarterly, 51*(1), 1–28. https://doi .org/10.2189/asqu.51.1.1

Fraser, S. (Ed.). (1995). *The bell curve wars: Race, intelligence, and the future of America.* Basic Books. ISBN 978-0-465-00693-9

Gardner, H. (1999). *Intelligence reframed: Multiple intelligences for the 21st century.* Basic Books.

Gladwell, M. (2011). *Outliers: The story of success.* Little, Brown and Co.

Goleman, D. (1995). *Emotional intelligence: Why it can matter more than IQ.* Bantam Books.

Haggbloom, S. J., Warnick, R., Warnick, J. E., Jones, V. K., Yarbrough, G. L., Russell, T. M., Borecky, C. M., McGahhey, R., Powell III, J. L., Beavers, J., & Monte, E. (2002). The 100 most eminent psychologists of the 20th century (PDF). *Review of General Psychology, 6*(2), 139–152. https://doi.org/10.1037/1089-2680.6.2.139

Healthfield, S. (2019). 360 degree feedback: See the good, the bad, and the ugly. *The Balance Careers.* https://www.thebalancecareers.com/360-degree -feedback-information-1917537

Hodzic, S., Scharfen, J., Ripoll, P., Holling, H., & Zenasni, F. (2017). How efficient are emotional intelligence trainings: A meta-analysis. *Emotion Review, 10*(2), 138–148. https://doi.org/10.1177/1754073917708613

Joseph, D. L., Jin, J., Newman, D. A., & O'Boyle, E. H. (2015). Why does self-reported emotional intelligence predict job performance? A meta-analytic investigation of mixed EI. *Journal of Applied Psychology, 100*(2), 298–342. https://doi.org/10.1037/a0037681

Joseph, D. L., & Newman, D. A. (2010). Emotional intelligence: An integrative meta-analysis and cascading model. *Journal of Applied Psychology, 95*(1), 54–78. https://doi.org/10.1037/a0017286

King, I. (1981). *A theory for nursing: Systems, concepts, processes.* Delmar Publishers, Inc.

Kotsou, I., Mikolajczak, M., Heeren, A., Grégoire, J., & Leys, C. (2019). Improving emotional intelligence: A systematic review of existing work and future challenges. *Emotion Review, 11*(2), 151–165. https://doi.org/10.1177/17540 73917735902

Martins, A., Ramalho, N., & Morin, E. (2010). A comprehensive meta-analysis of the relationship between emotional intelligence and health. *Personality and Individual Differences, 49*(6), 554–564. https://doi.org/10.1016/j.paid.2010.05.029

Mattingly, V., & Kraiger, K. (2019). Can emotional intelligence be trained? A meta-analytical investigation. *Human Resource Management Review, 29*(2), 140–155. https://doi.org/10.1016/j.hrmr.2018.03.002

Mayer, J. D., Caruso, D. R., & Salovey, P. (1999). Emotional intelligence meets traditional standards for an intelligence. *Intelligence, 27*(4), 267–298. https://doi.org/10.1016/S0160-2896(99)00016-1

Mayer, J. D., Caruso, D. R., & Salovey, P. (2016). The ability model of emotional intelligence: Principles and updates. *Emotion, 8*(4), 290–300. https://doi.org/10.1177/1754073916639667

Mayer, J. D., Salovey, P., Caruso, D. R., & Sitarenios, G. (2003). Measuring emotional intelligence with the MSCEIT V2. 0. *Emotion, 3*(1), 97–105. https://doi.org/10.1037/1528-3542.3.1.97

O'Boyle Jr., E. H., Humphrey, R. H., Pollack, J. M., Hawver, T. H., & Story, P. A. (2011). The relationship between emotional intelligence and job performance: A meta-analysis. *Journal of Organizational Behavior, 32*, 788–818. https://onlinelibrary.wiley.com/doi/abs/10.1002/job.714

Salovey, P., & Mayer, J. D. (1990). Emotional intelligence. *Imagination, Cognition, and Personality, 9*, 185–211.

Sánchez-Álvarez, N., Extremera, N., & Fernández-Berrocal, P. (2016). The relation between emotional intelligence and subjective well-being: A meta-analytic investigation. *The Journal of Positive Psychology, 11*(3), 276–285. https://doi.org/10.1080/17439760.2015.1058968

Schutte, N. S., Malouff, J. M., Thorsteinsson, E. B., Bhullar, N., & Rooke, S. E. (2007). A meta-analytic investigation of the relationship between emotional intelligence and health. *Personality and Individual Differences, 42*(6), 921–933. https://doi.org/10.1016/j.paid.2006.09.003

Sternberg, R. J., Forsythe, G. B., Hedlund, J., Horvath, J. A., Wagner, R. K., Williams, W. M., Snook, S. A., & Grigorenko, E. L. (2000). *Practical intelligence in everyday life.* Cambridge University Press.

Thorndike, E. L. (1920). Intelligence and its uses. *Harper's Magazine, 140*, 227–235. Cited in Landy, F. J. (2005). Some historical and scientific issues related to research on emotional intelligence. *Journal of Organizational Behavior, 26*, 411–424. https://doi.org/10.1002/job.317

Whpoteat.org (2020). William H. Poteat (1919–2020), philosopher.

2

The Anatomy and Physiology of Emotions

INTRODUCTION

Emotional skills are the heart of professional nursing. They are vital for patient assessment and effective nursing intervention. They are also indispensable for professional growth, leadership, team building, and self-care. This chapter seeks a deeper understanding of emotions themselves, of both their anatomy (the structure and function of emotions) and their physiology (the way emotions relate to human physiology). This chapter begins with a description of the nature of emotions and their physiological mechanisms. Emotional phenomena such as fight/flight, amygdalar hijacking, the relaxation response, and mind-body wellness are then described and explored. This chapter concludes with an introduction to the physiology of emotions as it relates to emotional intelligence ability.

THE PERIODIC TABLE OF THE EMOTIONS

From across the wide spaces of the British Library entryway, the large art piece on the far wall at first looked like the periodic table of the elements. On closer examination, it was titled, "The Periodic Table of the Emotions." Instead of C for carbon, C stood for Compassion; instead of Ag for argon, Ag was for anger. As well as being a clever piece of art, it carried a message: emotions are elemental. For nurses, this message has particular importance as they care for patients, interdisciplinary team members, and themselves.

Emotions Defined

What are emotions? Some experts define them as physiological phenomena, others as social and evolutionary ones. Are emotions the by-product

TABLE 2.1 Emotions Defined

DEFINITION	AUTHOR	PHILOSOPHICAL APPROACH	EXEMPLAR
Emotions are universal, an adaptive response to the environment	Darwin (1841)	Evolutionary: Emotions are universal	5 universal emotions (facial expressions in babies)
Emotions are physiological to experience	James-Lang (1994)	Physiological, "feelings" oriented	Different emotions have different physiology
Emotions are social phenomena that serve social purposes	Averill (1980)	Social constructivist	Emotional expressions vary among cultures
Cognitive and emotional elements of emotions are experienced simultaneously	Connan (1929)	Cognitive/ behaviorist	Physiological and subjective experiences are separate
Emotions are a cognitive phenomena	Arnold (1960)	Cognitive/ appraisal	Emotions are action tendencies
Emotions result from a combination of physiological and cognitive processes	The Schachter-Singer Theory (1962)	Cognitive	Physiological changes are noticed, then interpreted by environmental cues
Emotions exist within the context of the body-mind	Benson (2020)	Genetic/biological systems within bio-psycho-social-spiritual context	Relaxation response as a function of body-mind integration
Emotions are integrated from body, sensation, cognition, and action	Izard (1992)	Bio-psycho-social context	Emotions organize consciousness

Sources: Arnold, M. B. (1960). *Emotion and personality: Psychological aspects* (Vol. 1). Columbia University Press; Averill, J. R. (1980). A constructivist view of emotion. In *Theories of Emotion* (pp. 305–339). Academic Press. https://doi.org/10.1016/B978-0-12-558701-3.50018-1; Benson, H. (2020). *Mind Body Institute*. https://www.bensonhenryinstitute.org/about-us-dr-herbert-benson/; Cannon, W. B. (1929). *Bodily changes in pain, hunger, fear, and rage*. Appleton-Century-Crofts; Darwin, C., Ekman, P., & Prodger, P. (1998). *The expression of the emotions in man and animals*, 3rd ed. HarperCollins Publishers.; Izard, C. E. (1992). Basic emotions, relations among emotions, and emotion-cognition relations. *Psychological Review, 99*(3), 561–565. https://doi.org/10.1037/0033-295X.99.3.561; Izard, C. E. (2007). Basic emotion, natural kinds, emotional schemas, and a new paradigm. *Perspectives on Psychological Science, 2*(3), 260–280. https://doi.org/10.1111/j.1745-6916.2007.00044.x; Izard, C. E., Kagan, J., & Zajonc, R. B. (1984). *Emotions, cognition, and behavior*. Cambridge University Press, p. 17.; Lang, P. J. (1994). The varieties of emotional experience: A meditation on James-Lange Theory. *Psychological Review, 101*(2), 211–221. https://doi.org/10.1037/0033-295x.101.2.211; Schachter, S., & Singer, J. (1962). Cognitive, social, and physiological determinants of emotional state. *Psychological Review, 69*(5), 379–399. https://doi.org/10.1037/h0046234

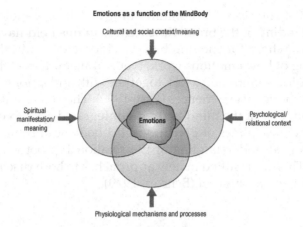

FIGURE 2.1 Emotions as a function of the Mind/Body.
Source: Adapted from Benson, H. (1979). *The mind/body effect: How behavioral medicine can show you the way to better health*. Simon & Schuster.

of physiological changes or vice versa? Does consciousness create emotions or is it the other way around? A range of approaches is summarized in Table 2.1.

In this text, emotions are conceptualized as bio-psycho-social-spiritual phenomena. They are "organized responses involving physical changes, felt experiences, cognitions and action plans, all with a strong evaluative component" (Izard, 2007, p. 260). The mind-body is the inseparable and deeply integrated relationship of human physiology, emotions, and cognition, a concept formulated by Herbert Benson, longtime physiology researcher on the relationship of the body and mind, and current director of Harvard's Mind/Body Institute (Benson, 2020) (see Figure 2.1).

Emotions are functions of the mind-body and within that integrated system, they organize consciousness.

EMOTIONS AND THE BODY

Physiologically, emotions involve the function of the cerebral cortex, structures under the cortex, and parts of the brain responsible for processing sensory information, such as the visual cortex. Emotional abilities depend on normal functioning of these structures. For example, research findings show lower measured emotional intelligence (EI) in people with lower-than-normal cortical function (Craig et al., 2009). For many years, the physiological understanding of emotions was restricted to the bioelectrical functions of nerves and hormones communicating between those structures.

The new field of psychoneuroimmunology (PNI), expanded this structural understanding of the brain. Researchers in this field have identified neuropeptides whose functioning has provided a dramatically different understanding of how emotions work. Neurotransmitters and hormones, these "molecules of emotion," work together with and among brain structures during emotional experiences (Pert, 1999). They constitute the physiological foundation of the mind-body the integrated system of body and mind. The new disciplines of PNI and mind-body science have also dramatically changed understanding of the relationship between emotions and disease. This has resulted in new approaches to both disease management and wellness promotion (Benson, 1979).

The Body in Love

The physiological changes of a person in love illustrate this interconnected web of brain structures, neurochemicals, and hormones. The physiological aspect is only one in the wondrous bio-psycho-social-spiritual phenomena of being in love, but it demonstrates the role of physiology in an emotional phenomenon. From a physiological standpoint, being in love has three general stages.

In the first stage, the social desire for romantic connection "primes the pump" by activating the hormones testosterone and estrogen. Upon meeting a romantic prospect, parts of the brain that perceive potential threats or stress are activated. As a result, the stress hormone cortisol is secreted. Not all stress is negative; the challenge of meeting an exciting person is stressful, albeit in a positive way. Increased cortisol levels have several physiological and emotional effects familiar to anyone in love—the beating heart, the sweaty palms! Initially, serotonin is suppressed. Emotionally this produces a preoccupation with, and intrusive thoughts about, the "object of romantic interest." Other chemical changes result in feelings of both euphoria and terror as soaring hopes and fears of rejection often accompany new love. At this point phenylethylamine (PEA), a stimulant, is secreted. This hormone causes the release of norepinephrine and dopamine. The effects of dopamine include elation, loss of mental focus, and heightened emotional sensitivity and reactivity. The "head over heels" feeling is quite physiological! These symptoms are also characteristic of addiction. The physiological changes in these two phenomena, early love and addiction, are identical (Breuning, 2015; Helmenstein, 2020; Schwartz & Olds, 2020).

A 2005 study of 2,500 students in love were shown pictures of their love interest. Their MRI scans were compared with ones accompanied by visualizations of casual acquaintances or friends. When shown pictures of loved ones, but not when looking at friends or acquaintances, particular regions of the brain demonstrated increased blood flow and chemical activity. These regions of the brain, including the caudate nucleus and the ventral tegmental area, are dopamine-rich structures. This neurotransmitter, sometimes called the "feel-good" chemical, creates euphoria, enhanced desire, and a focus on positive pleasure (Craig et al., 2009).

The caudate nucleus is also the "reward detection" center for the brain. It weaves together sensory information and social behavior to anticipate and recognize "rewards" such as various kinds of pleasure (food, love, sex). The ventral tegmental area of the brain is also related to pleasure, more specifically the motivation and behavior necessary to pursue and acquire pleasure rewards. These brain centers work in concert with other brain structures (amygdala, hippocampus, prefrontal cortex) to create a reward circuit, a self-reinforcing cycle that results in pleasure. At the same time, amygdalar (fight/flight) responses are diminished, suppressing fear, anxiety, and sadness. The combination of an activated pleasure–reward circuit and a suppression of fight/flight responses creates a sense of security in the early stages of being in love. Mid and frontal cortex function is also suppressed, decreasing use of logic, critical processes, and clear thinking (Schwartz & Olds, 2020). In this stage, literally, "love is blind."

In the second stage of being in love, the brain gradually develops a tolerance to the chemical changes from the first stage, but as the relationship develops and emotional attachment begins, other changes occur. Physical touch, even holding hands or casual social touching, stimulates oxytocin. Endorphins promote bonding and emotional experiences of contentment, calm, a sense of security, and reduced anxiety and stress. Serotonin, previously suppressed, surges. This increase is associated with elevated mood and positive emotions, but the opiate effects also create emotional dependency. In the third stage, as the relationship continues to develop over time, vasopressin, associated with long-term monogamy, becomes elevated (Breuning, 2015; Helmenstein, 2020; Schwartz & Olds, 2020).

This example illustrates why an understanding of the biochemical foundation for emotional experience is important in nursing practice. A patient comes to a nurse practitioner's clinic complaining of sleeplessness, palpitations, and obsessive thinking. Is it a cardiac condition, an anxiety disorder, or a new love? Identifying emotions accurately and understanding them depends on an understanding of the physiology of emotions and emotional responses. To identify and understand emotions, we must become, in the wonderful words of Dr. Mark Brackett, director of the Yale EI Laboratory, an "emotions scientist" (Brackett, 2019). This begins with understanding emotions better.

PHYSIOLOGICAL/EMOTIONAL PHENOMENA

Fight/Flight

In 1920, American physiologist Walter Cannon identified a series of physiological events in the body that occurred in threatening circumstances (Cannon, 1929). First named the fight/flight response, now more generally fight/flight/freeze these physiological changes are a response to activation of the sympathetic nervous system. They are now considered the first stage of response to acute stress, as described by Hans Selye's general adaptation syndrome (Selye, 1955). The physical fight/flight responses occur as a result of sympathetic nervous stimulation and adrenalin secretion. Fight/flight evolved in early humans as an emergency response.

Consider an early human's confrontation with a saber-toothed tiger. An adrenalin dump and sympathetic nervous system activation rapidly result in increased heart rate, blood pressure, cardiac output, and respiratory rate, all designed to enhance physical activity, strength, and physical capability. Muscle strength increases in preparation for physical confrontation. Increased nerve conduction speed makes sudden emergency movement easier. The voice becomes louder than usual to alert others and intimidate the threat. The visual field expands to take in dangerous changes in the environment. The entire physiology changes to prepare to fight the tiger or to flee. Blood shifts from relatively expendable extremities to central vital organs like the heart, lungs, and brain. Respiratory rate and lung capacity increase to make oxygen more available. The oxyhemoglobin dissociation curve shifts, facilitating release of oxygen from hemoglobin molecules into cells. Preparing for possible hemorrhage, blood coagulation rate increases and kidneys resorb water in case it is needed in the event of blood loss. Recall of information and taking in new data becomes more rapid.

The body does not distinguish between the stress of a saber-toothed tiger confrontation with the stress of a difficult interpersonal encounter. The physiological changes are the same. The body's response to an emotional threat in a social encounter is the same as if it were a physical threat. This is important to understand because strong emotions, particularly those related to safety (anger, fear, frustration, anxiety), trigger this physiological response (Jansen et al., 1995).

Amygdalar Hijacking

Another brain structure, the amygdala, is also involved in processing emotions related to survival. It mediates emotions like anger and fear, but also memory storage and retrieval. Potent memories and strong emotions are thought to be evoked by amygdalar function. Neuroscientist Joseph E. LeDoux demonstrated that, in some cases, emotional information moved from the thalamus, which receives and processes stress-related information, to the amygdala directly without engaging higher cognitive brain function. This results in powerful, rapid, and very strong emotional reactions. People who experience this physiological phenomenon often later report their reactions as being out of proportion to the situation that triggered the emotional response (Cunic, 2019). "I wasn't thinking" a person might say as if the emotions "took over," bypassing normal reasoning. Physiologically, that is exactly what occurred. Dr. Daniel Goleman named this phenomenon "amygdalar hijacking" (Goleman, 1995). "Triggered" emotions are often processed this way when powerful memories create strong emotional responses unmoderated by reasoning.

The Relaxation Response

Forty years after the identification of fight/flight physiology, Herbert Benson, another American physiologist at Harvard University, investigated physiological responses to emotions. He identified a collection of physiological responses that were the opposite of fight/flight, including lowered heart rate, lowered blood pressure and respiratory rate, muscle relaxation, and decreased alertness. He named this the "relaxation response," defining it as the "ability to encourage your body to release chemicals and brain signals that make your muscles and organs slow down and increase blood flow to the brain" (Benson, 1979, p. 26). Unlike the involuntary fight/flight response, the relaxation response can be intentionally elicited. Research has established the effectiveness of activities that elicit the relaxation response. Practices like deep breathing, meditation, yoga, and a variety of spiritual practices generate a relaxation response and have been used successfully to treat stress-related health problems. Research has shown they also effectively treat diseases that result from chronic stress, such as gastrointestinal dysfunction, high blood pressure, anxiety, and fibromyalgia. The relaxation response also has positive wellness benefits. More than 50 years of research has shown these practices to be associated with better health, lower blood pressure, heart rate, and stress levels, as well as higher levels of overall wellness (Mitchell, 2013).

EMOTIONAL PHYSIOLOGY AND EMOTIONAL INTELLIGENCE

EI is defined as the "ability to recognize the meanings of emotions and their relationships, and to reason and problem-solve on the basis of them" (Mayer et al., 1999, p. 267). EI is operationalized in the following abilities:

1. Accurate identification of emotions in self and others
*2. Understanding emotions
*3. Using emotions to reason
4. Managing emotions in oneself and emotional situations.
(Mayer et al., 1999).

*In this text, the second and third abilities are reversed from their usual order, as this order aligns better with the nursing processes illustrated throughout this work. Each of the four EI abilities draw upon, and are informed by, the emotional physiology of the mind-body.

Identifying Emotions Accurately and Understanding Emotions

Identifying emotions accurately enables the thoughtful "emotion scientist" to include an understanding of physiological phenomena in emotional problem-solving. For example, any emotion that activates adrenalin release (fight/flight or an amygdalar hijack) has the quality of an emergency.

These emotional responses in the body feel like an emergency because they are the physiological responses that prepare us for emergencies! This serves a human well when presented with a saber-toothed tiger in the backyard, but not as well in a conflict with a coworker. Again, the same physiological response occurs in interpersonal conflict that occurs with physical threats. The body cannot distinguish between them. The interpersonal conflict also feels like an emergency, which is why such conflicts so often escalate. By knowing when a person is in the throes of fight/flight, they could choose to slow down this emergency response. "I am too upset to talk with you right now. Let me take a walk then get back to you." Identifying "adrenalin-fueled" emotions in others is also crucial. Identifying that a coworker is angry and therefore physiologically engaged in a fight/flight please response will help interact with them more effectively. If instead the response is to "fight back," the interaction only gets worse. Two people in the chemical throes of fight/flight perceiving each other as a threat, can make resolving conflict difficult.

Using Emotions to Reason

First, identify an emotion. The emotion scientist in each of us can use this identification. "Oh! I am experiencing one of those adrenalin emotions!" Next, understand that emotion. "Okay. Anxiety is an adrenalin emotion.

Adrenalin emotions signal an emergency even when there isn't an emergency." As the face flushes, heart pounds, and the emotional pressure (emergency!) arises, understanding can be used to choose different behaviors.

This identification can help us use what we know about these emotions. It might look like this: "I feel like this is an emergency, and from the adrenalin, I might be agitated, red-faced, talk too loudly, and I might be emotionally confrontational. Knowing it is not really an emergency, I can choose a different response."

Managing Emotions in Oneself and in Emotional Situations

With this kind of "self-talk," a person can choose different behavior. Once they identify and understand "emergency emotions," and use them to reason, a person can manage emotions and emotional situations with better finesse. Is my voice too loud? Lower my voice. Am I hopping around the room in an agitated manner? Sit down and make eye contact. Am I having a general emergency reaction? Take a breath and a time out, maybe a quick walk outside, before I take the next step. To another person with us, we might say, "I am really anxious right now. Let me calm down a little and we can talk more later." Being specific, both to ourselves and to others, about emotions improves our communication.

NURSES AS EMOTION SCIENTISTS

Dr. Marc Brackett, one of the early EI researchers, suggested that people seek to be an "emotion scientist." This idea is inspirational and worth returning to again and again, particularly as the various chapters explore the development of EI ability.

> *Emotion scientists are curious, inquisitive, and analytical. They are active listeners and focus on facts. They ask people how they're feeling and really want to know. They listen well and pay careful attention to others' words and actions. They think long and hard about their own emotions too, always seeking to better understand their own emotional lives. They attempt and evaluate different ways of handling their emotions through trial and error.*

> (BRACKETT, *2019*).

This book is an invitation for nurses to be emotion scientists. This chapter began with an image to inspire that work, the "Periodic Table of the Emotions." This chapter ends with another image, a "Periodic Table of Emotions for Nurses" (Figure 2.2). An imagination exercise only, this challenges nurses to think about the emotions that are of particular interest in the specialty area in which they work.

	Burnout emotions						Self-Care emotions	
Obnoxious	Despair						Hope	
Sad	Hopelessness						Optimism	
Panic	Pessimism						Curiosity	
Disgust	Negativity						Passion	
Repulsed	Blaming	Neonatal and OB	ICU nursing	Oncology nursing			Gratitude	Understanding
Rejected	Judging	Equanimity	Determination	Hopeful	Easy-going	Relaxed	Happy	Happy
Hate	Irritation	Surprise	Fear	Anger	Sadness	Joy	Loving	Playful
Shame	Nervous	Confident	Shock	Shock	Quiet	Desire	Confident	Delight
Exhaustion	Insecurity	Grounded	Engagement	Denial	Cheery	Pride	Peaceful	Bubbly
Obnoxious	Depression	Tranquil	Excitement	Acceptance	Blissful	Trusting	Connected	Sympathy
Doubt	Frustration	Courage	Energy	Detachment	Kind	Ease	Bonded	Empathy
Envy	Fatigue	Capable	Elation	Acceptance	Trusting	Calm	Authentic	Compassionate

FIGURE 2.2 The periodic table of nurses' emotions.

DEVELOPING EMOTIONAL INTELLIGENCE

SAMPLE EMOTIONAL INTELLIGENCE DEVELOPMENT EXERCISE #1: MANAGING AMYGDALAR HIJACKING

Amygdalar hijacking is a scary experience. It feels out of control and often engages emotions that are unpleasant and difficult to deal with, including embarrassment. The EI abilities can help! First, identify the hijack! Recognizing that it is taking place is much of the work. Next, understanding that the emergency sensation that the hijacking involves is part of fight/flight. This then helps use that understanding to think about the situation. Slowing down the racing thoughts created by the hijack and fight/flight is important. It takes a few minutes for the fight/flight chemicals to clear the body. Use this time to evoke the relaxation response. Some deep breathing may help. Change locations. Move slowly. Disengage with others if possible to give yourself time to reflect. What happened? What triggered the hijack? Reflection breaks the hijack, reengaging the neocortex. Noticing memories and negative thoughts or fears might be especially helpful. Don't forget to recognize the positive aspects of the situation. What was learned and how the skill at managing the hijack changed can help restore a sense of control and balance (Cunic, 2019).

Source: Cunic, A. (2019). *Amygdala Hijack and the fight or flight response.* Very-Well. https://www.verywellmind.com/what-happens-during-an-amygdala -hijack-4165944

REFERENCES

Arnold, M. B. (1960). *Emotion and personality: Psychological aspects* (Vol. 1.). Columbia University Press.

Averill, J. R. (1980). A constructivist view of emotion. In *Theories of emotion* (pp. 305–339). Academic Press. https://doi.org/10.1016/B978-0-12-558701-3 .50018-1

Benson, H. (1979). *The mind/body effect: How behavioral medicine can show you the way to better health.* Simon & Schuster.

Benson, H. (2020). *Mind Body Institute.* https://www.bensonhenryinstitute.org/ about-us-dr-herbert-benson/

Brackett, M. (2019). *Permission to feel.* Macmillan.

Breuning, L. G. (2015). *Habits of a happy brain: Retrain your brain to boost your serotonin, dopamine, oxytocin, & endorphin levels.* F+W Media.

Cannon, W. B. (1929). *Bodily changes in pain, hunger, fear, and rage.* Appleton -Century-Crofts.

Craig, Y., Tran, Y., Hermens, G., Williams, L. M., Kemp, Y., Morris, C., & Gordon, E. (2009). Psychological and neural correlates of emotional intelligence in a large sample of adult males and females. *Personality and Individual Differences, 46*(2), 111–115. https://doi.org/10.1016/j.paid.2008.09.011

Cunic, A. (2019). *Amygdala Hijack and the fight or flight response.* VeryWell. https:// www.verywellmind.com/what-happens-during-an-amygdala-hijack-4165944

Darwin, C., Ekman, P., & Prodger, P. (1998). *The expression of the emotions in man and animals* (3rd ed.). Harper Collins Publishers.

Goleman, D. (1995). *Emotional intelligence: Why it can matter more than IQ.* Bantam Books.

Helmenstein, A. M. (2020). *Chemicals that make you feel love.* ThoughtCo. https://www.thoughtco.com/the-chemistry-of-love-609354

Izard, C. E. (1992). Basic emotions, relations among emotions, and emotion-cognition relations. *Psychological Review, 99*(3), 561–565. https://doi.org/10 .1037/0033-295X.99.3.561

Izard, C. E. (2007). Basic emotion, natural kinds, emotional schemas and a new paradigm. *Perspectives on Psychological Science, 2*(3), 260–280. https://doi.org/ 10.1111/j.1745-6916.2007.00044.x.

Jansen, A., Nguyen, X., Karpitsky, V., & Mettenleiter, M. (1995). Central command neurons of the sympathetic nervous system: Basis of the fight-or-flight response. *Science Magazine, 5236*(270), 644–646. https://doi.org/10.1126/science.270.5236.644

Kagan, J., & Zajonc, R. B. (1984). *Emotions, cognition, and behavior*. Cambridge University Press.

Lang, P. J. (1994). The varieties of emotional experience: A meditation on James–Lange Theory. *Psychological Review, 101*(2), 211–221. https://doi.org/10.1037/0033-295x.101.2.211

Mayer, J. D., Caruso, D., & Salovey, P. (1999). Emotional intelligence meets traditional standards for an intelligence. *Intelligence, 27,* 267–298. https://doi.org/10.1016/S0160-2896(99)00016-1

Mitchell, M. (2013). Dr. Herbert Benson's Relaxation Response Learn to counteract the physiological effects of stress. *Psychology Today.* https://www.floridamindfulness.org/resources/Documents/The%20Relaxation%20Response.pdf

Pert, C. B. (1999). *Molecules of emotion: The science behind mind-body medicine*. Simon & Schuster.

Schachter, S., & Singer, J. (1962). Cognitive, social, and physiological determinants of emotional state. *Psychological Review, 69*(5), 379–399. https://doi.org/10.1037/h0046234

Schwartz, K., & Olds, J. (2020). *On the brain: Love and the brain*. Newsletter of Harvard Medical School. https://neuro.hms.harvard.edu/harvard-mahoney-neuroscience-institute/brain-newsletter/and-brain/love-and-brain

Selye, H. (1955). Stress and disease. *Science, 122*(3171), 625–631. https://doi.org/10.1126/science.122.3171.625

3

Emotional Intelligence: The Nurse–Patient Relationship

INTRODUCTION

This chapter uses the ability emotional intelligence (EI) model as a framework to address the following questions:

1. Why is EI important in a nurse–patient relationship?
2. What do EI abilities look like in the care of patients?
3. What is the nursing research evidence for use of EI abilities in patient care?
4. Can nurse EI be developed?

In this chapter, these questions are used to explore the use of EI abilities to understand, evaluate, and improve clinical nursing practice.

APPLYING EI TO THE NURSE–PATIENT RELATIONSHIP: INTRODUCTION

Story: Active Shooter

The nurse was glued to the TV.

For days, an active shooter situation had left the city gripped in fear. Nobody knew if there was one or several shooters. Several people had been shot and killed. The city was living on edge. Commuting and daily life changed for everyone. Finally, a sniper had been found, cornered, shot by the police, and taken into custody.

On the live TV coverage, a medic unit loaded the wounded sniper into an ambulance and set off, sirens blaring and lights flashing.

Many conflicting emotions flooded the nurse, watching as reporters followed the medic unit to the yet undisclosed hospital. Anger, relief, and anxiety. Were there other shooters out there? Was the nightmare finally over?

On the screen, the medic unit turned off the freeway, onto the grounds of this nurse's hospital, taking the sniper to this nurse's ER, to this nurse's colleagues. The nurse, who oversaw safety protocols at the hospital, turned off the TV and headed for the ER.

What was going to happen next was important—critically important—on so many levels. Could the care the sniper receive affect the city's safety? Yes, because information was needed about whether the sniper had acted alone or had partners waiting to inflict further injury. How nurses interacted with the sniper emotionally could make gathering critical information easier or more difficult. Would the staff be challenged in their efforts to deliver professional, ethical, and appropriate care? Yes, particularly because of the damage their patient had caused and the terror he inflicted. Could the experience of caring for this person affect every nurse involved, even with the potential for long-term harm? Yes. Could this experience affect staff morale, stress, turnover, and professional commitment? From decades of research we know, the answer is yes. Could it also have the power to infuse the same nurses with deeper knowledge, wisdom, and professional grace? From the research we know, yes.

Applying EI Abilities

The case for nurse wisdom and expertise with emotional processes is not theoretical. Ample research evidence demonstrates its importance for patient outcomes and nurse self-care. Accurate identification of emotions in one's self and others, understanding emotions, using emotions to reason, and managing them in oneself and in emotional situations are core competencies required in every aspect of nursing practice. This is never more important than in the relationship between nurse and patient. Several principles guide this approach.

Emotional Intelligence Is Like CPR

Emotional intelligence (EI) abilities do not require a psychology degree or advanced training. Instead they are a bit like CPR. It does not take a physician to do CPR. It takes someone who has learned CPR, practiced it, and then uses the skills when needed. Emotional intelligence is like that. A person learns these abilities, practices them, and uses them when necessary. There is one big difference, though, between EI and CPR. No one does CPR not knowing they are doing CPR! But a lot of people, including many great nurses, use EI abilities all the time without being aware of it. The work of great nurses and brilliant clinical practice stories illustrate the use of EI abilities. In the evaluation of clinical errors and poor outcomes, it is also easy to identify the EI abilities that were not used.

Nurses who use EI abilities "naturally" are often not aware of the skills they are using. As with other skills, EI abilities can be evaluated and improved with intention and practice. Nursing skills of all kinds can be developed and EI ability is no exception. What about the people who do not have these abilities in their skill set? Many nurses resonate with the concept but just have not learned about EI. These nurses are ready to learn the language for describing EI and skill sets that EI ability represents.

Nurses' comfort with these skills varies with culture and family dynamics. Some people grow up in a family where feelings are respected as facts. They are negotiable facts that change quickly and evolve, but they are considered to be facts. These families employ language to describe and discuss feelings, and they commonly do so. In other cultures and other families, the lack of emotional expression and inadequate language to describe or discuss emotion is more typical. Nurses from varied emotional backgrounds are often excited to learn about the way EI ability helps them become "emotion scientists" who can identify, understand, use, and manage emotions better, and do emotional problem-solving, more effectively.

Some nurses disengage from emotional interaction with patients. They seem to wear an invisible t-shirt that says, "They don't pay me to care." Emotional distance, low levels of commitment, professional disengagement, lack of caring, and poor teamwork often characterize these nurses. But nurses are paid to care. It is a persistent myth that it is okay for some nurses not to care. But emotional labor is one kind of labor that is required of the job. Emotional abilities including emotional problem-solving are required to do nursing work. These abilities are not optional. This set of skills must be identified clearly and included in performance evaluation. The EI abilities offer a framework and specific definitions that enable nurses to do this.

Story: What Are You Doing?

The late 1970s saw one of the first research studies on nurse work, on what nurses actually *do*. A researcher in a grey suit carrying a clipboard followed nurses around their clinical unit for days, logging the nurses' activities, measured in minutes. At one point, one of the nurses stopped for a moment, gazing briefly at the ceiling.

Puzzled, the researcher asked, "What are you doing?"

The nurse answered truthfully, "I was thinking."

The researcher looked at the nurse, at the clipboard, and back at the nurse. "I don't have a category for that."

Story Reflection

Nursing has come a long way. The profession now has a deep lexicon about nurse thinking. Nurses are interested in both cognitive and physical labor and recently have added emotional labor to this list. The negative impact of emotional labor, manifested in compassion, fatigue, and caregiver exhaustion, is now a major subject of discussion. The profession now grapples with the fiscal, professional, and personal impact of emotional labor and the importance of understanding its effect on perceived stress, job performance, clinical patient outcomes, and nurse longevity. What the profession has yet to do is operationalize elements of emotional labor. The EI ability model offers nurses a way to do this. It also offers the opportunity to make these concepts part of specific performance requirements.

IDENTIFYING EMOTIONS

APPLYING EI ABILITIES TO THE NURSE–PATIENT RELATIONSHIP

When it is just a nurse at the bedside, what do EI abilities look like? How are these abilities used in the nurse–patient relationship? How are the four EI abilities, identifying emotions, understanding them, using them to reason and managing, are applied to patient care (Mayer et al., 1999)? Note: in this chapter, their usual order is adapted to best align with the nursing process.

Using EI: Identifying Emotions Accurately

The foundational EI ability is accurate identification of emotions. Emotions are information! This skill involves accurate identification of the emotions in ourselves and other people. It is surprisingly easy to assume how someone else is feeling, only to find out how wrong this assumption was. If we are mistaken, the consequences can be serious, particularly in the healthcare setting. An example familiar to most nurses, the patient who looks angry, but is actually acutely frustrated, is diagrammed in Figure 3.1.

This diagram illustrates a situation in which a patient demonstrates behavior that includes a raised voice, confrontational demeanor, and aggressive words. The nurse, without confirming the patient's emotion, concludes the patient is angry. If the patient said, "I am so angry," the nurse could safely assume the patient is in fact angry, and develop and execute

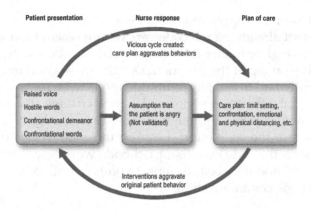

FIGURE 3.1 Inaccurate identification of an emotion: misidentification of anger.

a plan of care. Habitually angry, aggressive, or confrontational patients may need a plan of care that includes exploring the anger, setting limits on angry outbursts, and instituting measures to physically and emotionally protect the staff. But what if the nurse is wrong? Other feelings that hospitalized patients often experience, like fear and frustration, can look like anger. What if the patient is frightened or frustrated or emotionally overwhelmed? Figure 3.1 illustrates what could happen next.

If the nurse bases the plan of care on an incorrect assessment of an emotion, the patient's emotional condition could worsen. For example, isolating a patient (care plan for anger) could increase the real emotion: frustration. Figure 3.1 reflects the reinforcing feedback loop common in clinical practice. This vicious cycle can only be broken when the patient's feelings are correctly identified, and the plan of care modified. Without this basic emotional problem-solving, the plan of care does not work and other aspects of the patient's care such as trust in the care team can be compromised.

In contrast, if the nurse used another EI ability, understanding emotions, the outcome could be different. A simple question like, "Can you tell me more about what is going on?" could lead to correctly identifying the patient's emotions. The patient may be angry, and the nurse's clarifying question would communicate acceptance and validation. But if they are not, further discussion could help both the patient and nurse clarify the patient's true feelings and how the nurse can help. To further illustrate this, two clinical examples are used. The first illustrates the importance of identifying one's own feelings correctly, and the second illustrates how easy it is to misidentify patients' feelings.

Story: The First Code (Taking Your Own Pulse)

It was the nurse's first code. She was assigned to the code cart and was trying hard to pay attention to everything and to help as much as possible. Several times, when she was asked for something, she knew right where it was—in the supply room! She would run across the room to get what was in fact already on the code cart within reach. During the code, the nurse's voice grew louder and she talked a lot. She wanted to be perceived as being on top of the situation. Despite these good intentions, the nurse frequently had to ask for communications to be repeated.

After the code, the team performed a code critique. The team identified that the novice nurse, although obviously trying hard, had contributed confusion to the code effort. Leaving the code to get supplies that were actually on the code cart disrupted code workflow. Too much talking, loud voices, and the need for repeat communication had all contributed to poor code communication.

Story reflection

When the critical care instructor reviewed the code with the nurse, she recommended, "take your own pulse." This suggestion involved identifying emotions. In her desire to perform well, this anxious novice was supercharged physiologically by fight/flight. Psychologically, she was trying hard to perform well, but the resulting flood of fight/flight response neurotransmitters made her large muscles want to fight or flee … or to move across the room to get supplies already within reach. Hyper-verbal and loud voices also result from fight/flight anxiety. Her field of attention was very wide and unfocused (another physiological response to stress), so requests or directions had to be repeated. Understanding this physiological aspect of her emotion, the nurse was able to use her emotions to reason and problem-solve her code performance. Aware that her fight/flight responses negatively affected her code performance, she decided to follow her mentor's advice and make a habit of metaphorically "taking her own pulse." Identifying fight/flight emotions right away kept them from compromising her performance. In future codes, she became more mentally focused, quieter, and more physically still. In this case, correctly identifying her emotions accurately was the first step in improving her code performance.

Story: Don't Comfort Me!

Another example of correctly identifying emotions, this time the patient's emotions, is illustrated in the emergency hospitalization of a patient who was also a retired nurse. Although a relatively small event, it illustrates what can happen when a nurse does not identify an emotion correctly. Experiencing new onset chest pain for the first time after decades of good health, the patient, also a retired nurse, was transferred from a small rural hospital to a tertiary center across the state. She endured repeated assessments across several hospitals, some by obvious novices. Finally, at the end of a horrific and anxiety-filled day, she received the good news that her workup revealed no serious problems. Having managed to stay calm all day, she finally lost it and cried. She had held it together all day on an emotional roller coaster. She had stayed patient with inexperienced nurses. When she finally received the good news that all test results had been negative, she was relieved beyond words. Hearing positive clinical news, the resulting letdown hit her all at once, and emotionally exhausted, she cried from sheer relief. Her nurse entered the room, saw the tears, and reached out, patting her on the shoulder and trying to comfort her, "There, there … all your tests are negative, don't worry."

This patient was not, in fact, worried at all. She had reviewed the EKG, lab work, and CT scan herself and knew to rule out an MI. She was relieved, tired, and in emotional letdown. She just needed a good cry. If asked, she would have requested to be left alone to quietly process the emotional events of the day. But her nurse did not correctly identify her emotions. Her misidentification of her patient's feelings disrupted the nurse–patient relationship. The interaction not only felt "off" to the patient, but also undermined trust in the nurse–patient relationship. The plan of care failed. The flow of this case study as it occurred is illustrated in Figure 3.2.

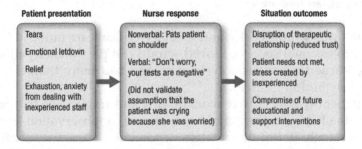

FIGURE 3.2 Misidentification of emotions: relief and letdown misidentified as worry.

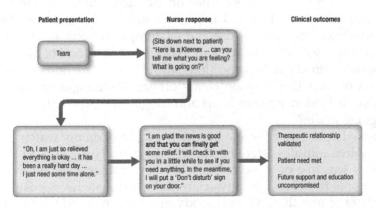

FIGURE 3.3 Accurate identification of emotions: identification of relief.

Figure 3.3 illustrates how EI ability can be used to correctly identify the patient's emotions. This changes the outcome.

Story Reflection

Identifying emotions correctly in oneself and in others and checking assumptions about what others are feeling can prevent not only miscommunication and misidentification of problems, but also inadvertent disruption of the caring relationship that is the foundation of the plan of care.

APPLYING EI ABILITIES: IDENTIFYING EMOTIONS ACCURATELY AND UNDERSTANDING EMOTIONS

The prior two stories focused on one EI ability, but EI abilities generally work together. This next example illustrates this.

Story: Regret, an Interview

To be fair, I was young, cocky, and a novice critical care nurse in the flush of early professional success. I loved what I did passionately, adored my patients, learned voraciously every day, and had more than a little ego riding on my budding career.

My patient was an elderly woman, tiny and fragile. She had been admitted to the ICU as a precautionary measure for observation. She never had been acutely ill but nonetheless needed close observation. She was stable and doing fine. She did not have transfer orders yet, but if we needed the bed, she would have been first to go.

I reported for my shift, saw her on my assignment, got the report, which was unremarkable, and began rounds on my patients. We had met before and there was a close and easy rapport between us. I was always fond of my elder patients, and I was especially fond of her. As I did rounds, she seemed oddly preoccupied and fretful. Patients often are after the shock of an ICU admission wears off and the danger nearly averted hits them. As I listened to her heart and lungs, she looked at me and said, 'Am I going to die?'

I looked at her cheerily and brightly said, 'Not on my watch!'

Forty-five minutes later she coded and died. Not just died but died awfully. It was one of those codes where everything goes wrong. Competent people fumbled. The physician had to intubate her repeatedly and the roof of her mouth was soon bloody and torn. As I did CPR and broke a rib for the first time, I silently prayed, 'Don't come back into this body, don't come back.'

Using EI: Identifying Emotions Accurately

Using EI to understand this situation, what went wrong other than the nurse's obvious and abject failure to do mouth control? How can EI be used to problem-solve this clinical disaster? Learning from this situation and moving forward, what could have been done differently? Also, how can EI abilities prevent post-error trauma and enhance professional resilience and professionalism?

The error cascade began when the nurse did not identify an emotion correctly. When the patient asked, "Am I going to die?" the nurse assumed she was having typical ICU anxiety. Being in ICU is scary. Patients realize they have been sick enough to be in ICU, so fear of death is common. Nonetheless, the patient's question should have been a red flag. It was out of character for this patient, who was not typically anxious, but the nurse did not register this emotional information as important data. She did not draw the patient out, ask questions, and make sure she correctly identified the emotion the patient was expressing. In this case, the patient's question was not a question but a statement. She was not fearfully asking if she would die. The patient asked the question calmly, almost matter of fact. There was no fear in her face or tone of voice. In retrospect, the nurse came to believe the patient was experiencing a premonition, an emotional perception, a warning.

Using EI: Understanding Emotions

The nurse did not use her understanding of emotions. Later, she reported she knew patients experience premonitions of danger. Very often, the first sign of an impending physiological crisis is an affective, emotional change in the patient. The patient's physiology has changed, registering danger. This was fundamental to intervening in this situation. The nurse did not identify the patient's emotions correctly or use her understanding of emotions to assess the patient correctly.

Story Reflection

This nurse was later asked to analyze her story, using EI abilities to rewrite the outcome. Identifying emotions accurately is not usually hard. A few questions need to be asked. Perceptions and assumptions need to be checked. She said, "If I could rewrite history, I would have put down my stethoscope, sat on my patient's bed, taken her hands in mine, looked in her eyes, and asked what was going on."

The nurse said, "That this patient's affect was out of character was information, a red flag. I could have used my understanding of premonitions to intervene differently. I would have taken her question seriously, hugged and reassured her. I would have told her I would check in with her often and perhaps encouraged her to call a friend. Maybe, I would have done some charting in her room or just, if I could have, hung out with her and chatted. Her death was probably not preventable but she might have died less scared."

APPLYING EI ABILITIES: USING EMOTIONS TO REASON AND MANAGING EMOTIONS

Story: Anger as Information

When emotions and reason are integrated instead of separated, thinking informs feeling and feeling informs thinking. This can be illustrated by the story of a nurse struggling in a relationship with her patient, a young man admitted for pain control after a car accident. An exceptionally caring nurse, known for her ability to bond with and support patients, she confessed she found herself perpetually and inexplicably angry with this patient. Confused and concerned about burnout or acting unprofessionally, she reached out to her mentor.

"Are there types of patients who tend to make you angry?" her mentor asked, suggesting the nurse see her anger as information. Sometimes anger is a reaction to a situation, but sometimes it is information about the situation itself.

"Oh, boy, yes!" she exclaimed. "I hate it when patients try to manipulate me, it makes me really crazy!" She laughed, but then stopped. In that moment, she was integrating her anger with what she knew about herself and anger. She was "think/feeling." She became conscious for the first time that her patient was, in fact, trying to manipulate her. This behavior was disguised by his superficially pleasant, gregarious, and emotionally engaging personality.

She talked with other nurses caring for him. A clear pattern emerged. The patient was playing staff against each other, trying to undermine the pain control plan whose goal was weaning him off narcotics.

Using EI: Using Emotions to Reason

Integrating feelings as data into thinking about the situation was crucial for working with this patient effectively. Once the nurse accepted her own feelings as "data" and understood the clinical implications, she had no difficulty returning to her patient with a more effective plan of care. By sharing what she had learned with the rest of the staff, others avoided falling into the emotional trap, and the staff's care of the patient became more effective.

Using EI: Managing Emotions

Once emotions are identified accurately and understanding of them is used to reason, then emotional problem-solving becomes more effective. EI is not about controlling or suppressing emotions, which is a tremendous drain of energy and often ineffective. For example, it is exhausting and pointless to try to not to be angry with someone you are in an argument with. If the response instead is, "I am really angry. Maybe I can use this energy to do something constructive, like solve the problem that made me angry?" In this case, repressing the anger could have eaten away the rest of the day. Accepting it and using the energy it generated could have a positive result.

Story: Regret Revisited (From an EI Application Exercise)

A patient's room after a code is hard to describe. The resuscitation team has left. Supplies and trash are strewn about. Someone has closed drapes and doors so other patients and family members are spared the sight. Two beings are left, one alive and one not, the nurse and the patient. Until the code, the patient had been stable. My other patient had not been and needed my attention. I was reeling with emotions, including sadness and guilt. To catalog my feelings in that moment would have taken more time than I had. Taking time to feel everything I needed to process the events would take weeks. My other patient needed me fully present and focused. Managing my feelings did not require denying them or trying to control them, but simply acknowledging their power. I would return to them when I had more time.

Using EI: Managing Emotions

My ritual helped me. I used it for self-care working in critical care where death was always close. I used it when my patient died or was close to death. I would say silently to myself, "Death, my old friend, what will you teach me this time?" That question was a promise to myself and to my patient that I would not rush past my feelings nor leave them unfelt. I would honor the patient and myself by returning to them, again and again. I would let them teach me, making me a better nurse, and a deeper, wiser person.

Story Reflection

As the nurse reflected on this story many years after the event, she wondered why this traumatic event in her professional life did not harm her, make her callous, or burned out. Ultimately, it made her a better nurse who loved nursing throughout her professional life. Although she did not know about EI back then, she later understood that identifying emotions, understanding them, using them to reason, and managing emotions benefitted her wellness, wisdom, and professional growth.

RESEARCH EVIDENCE: EI AND CLINICAL NURSING PRACTICE, AN IMPORTANT CONCEPT?

A basic review of the first 20 years of nursing research on EI is summarized in Chapter 15. In short, the first nursing EI research study was published in Portugal in 1999 and was followed over the next 20 years by the hundreds of published nursing research studies (dos Santos et al., 1999). The findings of these studies often were validated by the growing body of EI research from other disciplines. In those 20 years, nurse researchers from over 40 countries published evidence for relationships between EI and nurse clinical performance, retention on the job, nurse physical and mental health, team and leadership effectiveness, and positive patient outcomes.

The body of evidence continues to evolve, but the fundamental question, "Is EI is an important concept for nursing?" seems to have a clear answer. Based on the research science now available, the answer is unequivocally yes! Secondly to the question, "Is there a relationship between nurse EI and important clinical, organizational, and professional outcomes?" The answer is also clearly yes. Research evidence demonstrates a significant relationship between EI and clinical, organizational, and professional outcomes, including nurse performance, nurse perceived stress, emotional coping, and caring. Positive clinical outcomes, both physiological outcomes and those related to nurse caring, also correlate with nurse EI. There is also research evidence of correlation between EI and nurse retention, team effectiveness, and professional engagement. For further detail, description, and analysis of the research findings, see Chapter 15.

DEVELOPING EI ABILITY

A substantial body of research evidence in nursing and other disciplines supports the effectiveness of a wide range of activities to improve EI. A first step in developing EI ability is identifying each person's own, personal, individual, and constantly expanding menu of options to select from in order to manage an emotional situation. Like the ritual described in the last story, these practices help us to process emotions effectively and support the development and use of EI abilities.

Story: The Menu (From an EI Reflection Exercise)

Meg, one of my clinical students, came flying into my office one day, shortly after she had attended my class on EI. Without greeting or pleasantries, she announced abruptly "OK, I am a believer. I get emotional intelligence. What do I do now?"

I had to laugh. I knew Meg well enough to know when she decided to tackle something, she did it right away. "What are you working on?"

Meg explained that her friends often complained that when she was mad, she yelled at them. Yelling was her go-to response. She asked, "How can emotional intelligence help me?"

After encouraging her for taking this on, I reminded her that some emotions are fueled physiologically by adrenalin. Anger, fear, frustration, and panic feel similar and can be difficult to distinguish. They may masquerade as, and blend with, each other. Being focused on survival, they also feel like an emergency. It feels like you have to do something right away.

"But what else could I do? I am mad, I feel like I am going to explode. I just have to yell. What else could I do?" Meg asked.

Meg was no dummy, and later that day we would talk about saying things like, "Our relationship is really important to me, but right now I am too upset to talk. I will get back to you later." But in the moment, I simply said, "What if you just walked away?"

She looked stunned. Then she said clearly to herself , "I could walk away. I could walk away!" She got up, and without a word, left my office muttering, "I could walk away."

This moment in my office was shocking to her because she suddenly had not one but two things on her menu. By the end of the day, she had several perfectly acceptable other options that she could see herself doing instead of yelling at her friends.

DEVELOPING EMOTIONAL INTELLIGENCE ABILITY

EMOTIONAL INTELLIGENCE DEVELOPMENT SAMPLE EXERCISE #3: THE MENU

This idea of developing a menu of ways to manage difficult emotions and difficult situations is a great way to begin to develop emotional intelligence abilities. To do this, begin with some basic questions: What emotions are you good at? Which come easily? With which are you most comfortable? Which ones not so much? Which ones do you dislike or avoid? What situations or interactions with other people drive you crazy? One great way to begin developing ability is to think about your own menu, what works well for you, but also where your menu is thin or ineffective. Brainstorming possible additions to your menu and talking with others about what is on theirs is an excellent place to begin.

Source: Original to author

REFERENCES

dos Santos, L. M., de Almeida, F. L., & da Costa Lemos, S. (1999). Emotional intelligence: Testing the future nursing. *Revista Brasileira de Enfermagem, 52*(3), 401–412. https://doi.org/10.1590/s0034-71671999000300010

Mayer, J. D., Caruso, D., & Salovey, P. (1999). Emotional intelligence meets traditional standards for an intelligence. *Intelligence, 27*, 267–298. https://doi.org/10.1016/S0160-2896(99)00016-1

4

Emotional Intelligence: Caring for Patient Families, Colleagues, and Teams

INTRODUCTION

Nurses have discussed the importance of understanding emotional systems for many years. Hildegard E. Peplau and other theorists explicated the importance of effective communication not only for patient care but for successful practice within complex organizations (Freshwater & Stickley, 2004; King, 1981; Peplau, 1992). Imogene King's Interacting Systems Theory (IST), for example, posits personal, interpersonal, and social systems in constant and changing interaction, which provides the context for interaction among individuals, relationships, and groups. King's theory suggests nurses require skills to understand and navigate these systems, not only as they establish therapeutic relationships but throughout all aspects of the nursing process. However, the theory does not explicate those skills. The emotional intelligence (EI) abilities can easily make the skills outlined in King's conceptual theory specific and measurable (Shanta & Connoly, 2013). In this chapter, the four EI abilities, identifying emotions, understanding them, using them to reason and managing, are applied to care of families, colleagues and nurse teams. (Mayer et al., 1999). Their usual order is adapted to best align with the nursing process.

APPLYING EI ABILITIES TO NURSING THEORY

Identifying Emotions

King considered accurate identification of a patient's emotions as integral to supporting the patient to achieve health. Indeed she also emphasized this to prevent misperception of patient emotions. According to King, all aspects of both therapeutic communication and care planning depend upon fundamental accuracy in emotional assessment. At the same time, according to her theory, nurses must also identify their own emotions for their own wellness. Identifying emotions, the emotional intelligence (EI) ability on which all the others rest, operationalizes King's description of this dynamic (Shanta & Connoly, 2013).

Understanding Emotions

The interpersonal system component of IST, as it includes effective inter-actions and empathy, depends on effective communication, caring, and other interpersonal relationship skills. All these elements of clinical com-munication correlate with EI ability (see Chapter 14 for specific research findings). These elements also contribute to nurses' understanding of their own emotions and those of other people around them. EI research-ers Mayer and Salovey define empathy, arguably one of the core concepts for nursing, as the ability to understand the feelings of others. In this way, a second EI ability, understanding emotions, effectively operationalizes nurse functions within the IST interpersonal system.

Using Emotions to Reason

King's IST offers a theoretical framework for nursing that integrates cognition and emotions. It established using emotions to reason as a necessary skill to navigate the three interactional systems. Thus, using emotions to reason was suggested as a core skill for nursing years before it was described as a core EI ability.

Managing Emotions in Oneself and in Emotional Situations

The nursing process depends on EI abilities (Shanta & Connoly, 2013). Identifying EI abilities as an operationalization of the skills King's theory suggests (1) their role in therapeutic relationships, (2) their utility in the nursing process, and (3) their importance as mediators of caring, effective communication, rapport building, and interpersonal relationship skills. Research findings in nursing, as well as other disciplines, have shown that these abilities correlate with EI (for specific research findings, see Chapter 15).

Accurate assessment is the foundation for effective nursing interven-tions. EI ability supports accurate assessment in several ways. First, it helps create strong relationships with patients, fostering trust and effective communication. In this case, patients are more willing to tell the truth, helping nurses accurately assess the patient's problems, capabilities, and responses to treatment. EI abilities also enable nurses to integrate thinking and feeling to use emotions to reason, improving their clinical reasoning pathways. Nurses often talk about "bonding" with their patients. This indicates a strong emotional connection with the patient. When nurses do this, they are using their emotions to reason. The nursing process becomes an integrated phenomenon, weaving together thinking, feeling, and care planning. Some nurses refer to this as intuition, but it may instead be deep assessment, recognition of fact patterns, and a profound integration of body/mind/spirit assessment into care.

APPLYING EI ABILITIES TO CARE OF PATIENT'S FAMILIES

Story: Brains on the Pillow

With equal parts irreverence and resigned sadness, nurses in the trauma unit referred to this as a "brains on the pillow" situation. A young man had shot himself in the head, an inoperable, unsurvivable, and catastrophic injury. If there was such a thing as a trauma hospice unit, he would have been in it. There was little but supportive care left for this man and his family. Many trauma injuries take place within the context of complex family stories and this patient's certainly had. This young man had told his friends and coworkers he was gay years before. But when he eventually came out to his immediate family, his mother rejected him roughly. Distraught, he returned home and shot himself.

His mother now visited him daily. She was angry and loud, and she persistently criticized every aspect of her son's nursing care: the way the bed was made, failure to turn her son more frequently, the state of his nails, and when he was bathed last. She was hostile, belligerent, and unreachable. She rejected any compassion or support from the staff. She listened to the physician reports every day wordlessly, lips clenched, but upon the nursing staff she unleashed her wrath. Nothing penetrated her verbal wall of hostility and the staff had begun to avoid her.

A novice nurse orienting to the unit was assigned to assist in this patient's care. Early one day, she was unexpectedly accosted by the mother, already on a tirade. The novice nurse was completely thrown off-balance. No education or experience had prepared her for the verbal onslaught. She blurted, "Do you know this is not your fault?"

The patient's mother looked as if she had been slapped. She burst into tears and, sobbing uncontrollably, threw herself into the arms of the novice nurse. To the nurse's coworkers the sight was unforgettable, the look on the stunned novice's face, looking at her coworkers over the sobbing woman's shoulder, patting her back wordlessly.

This woman had not known her son's actions were not her fault. In fact, she was convinced they were, and she assumed the staff judged her harshly. In reality, her self-judgment and guilt were overwhelming. Much, much later, she would accept that while she would forever regret her actions, it had been her son's own decision to end his life. The novice's simple question was her first step on that long journey to healing.

Applying EI Abilities

How can this simple, seemingly miraculous, interaction be understood? The four EI abilities are easily recognized in the story.

Using EI: Identifying Emotions Accurately

Identifying emotions accurately in oneself and in others sounds easy, but this story illustrates how far this is from the truth. The patient's mother appeared angry, as suggested by her verbal and nonverbal behavior. If asked, "What are you feeling?" she would have likely identified anger as her primary feeling. Although the nurse in this story was a novice, she exemplified what an "emotion scientist" looks like. In a blink, she did not accept the "easy answer." She reached beyond it, past the wall of anger. Her refusal to accept the easy answer was a crucial step in emotional problem-solving.

Using EI: Understanding Emotions

Intense expressions of anger are often just what they appear to be, but it must be understood that anger is also often used as a defense mechanism. A person may use it to cope with other, more difficult or less socially acceptable, feelings. A family member who is terrified, frustrated, or feeling guilty may avoid these by expressing anger instead. When the intensity of anger seems either inappropriate (dirty nails on an essentially brain-dead patient) or out of proportion to the situation, something other than simple anger is probably going on.

This emotional information constitutes a "red flag." When anger's complexity is understood, you can look deeper into the emotion underneath it. When this is happening, anger is part of a coping mechanism. People use coping mechanisms because they need to, because they are in trouble. Anger used in this way is a cry for help.

Using EI: Using Emotions to Reason and Managing Emotions

The mother's terrible weight of guilt and self-judgment was redirected into anger at the staff. When a nurse correctly identifies an emotion, understands the emotion, and uses this information to reason, they can differently assess the situation and plan how to manage it. In this story, the nurse identified an emotion correctly and used her understanding of anger and guilt. She integrated understanding, thinking, and feeling to ask a short, simple question that changed everything.

Story Reflection

In this situation, the four EI abilities came together in a flash. If asked, the novice nurse likely would have chalked her actions up to impulse or intuition, as often nurses do. Nonetheless, this story illustrates how quickly and powerfully the four EI abilities can transform a challenging clinical situation.

APPLYING EI ABILITIES TO TEAM CONFLICT

Interdisciplinary conflict is among the biggest challenges for nurses. It also negatively impacts patient care, making it less effective and less safe.

Story: The Nurse-Doctor War

Every nursing team struggles with conflict between physicians and nurses at some time. It is destructive, decreases, morale, stifles learning, and inevitably compromises patient care.

On Unit 4 South, the conflict between nurses and physicians had grown steadily over years. Hearts hardened and relationships polarized to the point of paralyzing the interdisciplinary care team. Team rounds were impossible and even basic clinical interactions carried a negative emotional charge. As a solution, the physicians' staff tried to take control of the nursing team, undermining the nurse manager's authority, and attempted to replace her with the wife of one of the physicians, a nurse on the staff with no leadership experience. Medical and nursing care became essentially separate, parallel processes. Team members from other disciplines tiptoed around the conflict, trying not to get caught in the institutional crossfire. Care was compromised. Patients noticed the pervasive hostility and tension in the care team. Hospital administration tried to resolve the conflict by taking sides, supporting the physician staff. Nursing staff morale plummeted, and the nurse manager resigned. The unit nurse educator was asked to be the interim nurse manager. She had consulting experience and was skilled in conflict resolution and team care. It was hoped that she could at least stabilize the situation until a new nurse manager could be hired.

Applying EI Abilities

In a long-term conflict like this one, hurt feelings, miscommunication, misinterpretations, and misunderstandings over years often form layer after layer until the heaviness of half composted relationships renders the situation difficult to understand and impossible to navigate. The interim manager decided untangling the past was impossible. She focused on the present to find a way for the unit to move forward. This plan was fueled by necessity when hospital administration notified her that the unit was moving into a new wing of the hospital, about to begin construction. The interim manager would be responsible for leading the design and construction of the unit and for coordinating the transfer of patients, services, and staff.

Using EI: Identifying Emotions

Concerned about team dysfunction jeopardizing the entire effort, the interim manager had to first formulate her own assessment of the physician-nurse conflict and the overall team dysfunction. Then, she had to involve the whole team in the new unit design. As part of her orientation to the new role, she scheduled one-on-one meetings with nurses, physicians, members of other disciplines, administrators, and support staff. She started every conversation with a simple question: "How are you feeling these days about your work on the team?" She heard about hurt feelings and criticisms, but more importantly, about common feelings of frustration and embarrassment. Everyone knew the situation was ridiculous. There had been unprofessional behavior and power grabs on both sides. The consensus was it was time to move on and do better, but no one seemed to have an idea how. By identifying the emotional consensus of the group, the nurse manager had a place to begin.

Using EI: Understanding Emotions and Using Emotions to Reason

The interim nurse manager started by identifying the group frustration and embarrassment. She then used her understanding of typical group conflict emotions. She had to identify common ground for the unit to learn to work together. This understanding helped her use her emotions to reason through the next steps.

The key emotion she became aware of was frustrated paralysis. The group wanted to move forward, but they did not know how, so they stayed locked in the same familiar, destructive patterns. Her understanding of frustrated paralysis helped the nurse manager plan. This feeling does not respond well to education or instruction. It often requires something more basic. The staff, doctors, and nurses alike, had to be shown what to do.

Using EI: Managing Emotions

The interim nurse manager's understanding of frustrated paralysis enabled her to "think/feel" her way to the next step in managing the situation. If the team did not know how to take the first step, she was going to have to show them. Not tell them, not advise them, but show them. She found a physician with whom to partner, hoping such a partnership could build a bridge between the two groups and also show such partnership was possible.

The last thing the outgoing nurse manager had said was, "Watch out for Dr. Green. She is sneaky and can't be trusted. She is the real power in the physician group." Dr. Green was a brilliant woman who had not seemed overtly involved in the team conflict. She held no official role on the unit, so these words had seemed odd. On a hunch, the interim manager scheduled a coffee date with Dr. Green.

The meeting began awkwardly as the two women got to know each other. At first, they fell into the old pattern of finger-pointing and blame. But while talking about the ridiculousness of the situation and the immaturity on both sides, one of them started to laugh. The ice broke. The two mentally rolled up their sleeves and discussed the exciting possibilities the new construction and unit relocation offered. By the end of the meeting, they had decided to meet weekly. Moreover, they discovered in each other not only an able professional partner, but in the weeks and months ahead, a good friend.

The partnership between the two surprised both physicians and nurses. The interim manager had been known in her nurse educator role to be a fierce nurse advocate, and pretty much everyone on the unit expected her to adamantly retake control of the clinical operations on the unit, as was her responsibility. The physicians who had overstepped their role were surprised when the interim nurse manager immediately gave Dr. Green, representing the physician staff, time, access, and input into decisions about the new unit design and plans for the move. That meant their needs and priorities were going to have a strong advocate in Dr. Green. The physicians stepped back, relaxed, stopped micromanaging, and refocused on patient care.

The nurses, who saw Dr. Green as "the worst of the worst," could not believe the support Dr. Green gave their nurse manager. The nurses discovered, to their surprise, Dr. Green was advocating for them, helping the doctors to understand nursing staff issues. As plans for the new unit evolved, the interim nurse manager asked for volunteers for subgroups to help with various aspects of the planning and implementation of the new unit. Physicians and nurses were on all the teams. None of the staff, neither nurses nor physicians, had ever designed and built a clinical unit before. In their partnerships, nurses and doctors alike had to help each other, trust each other's skills and ideas, and take risks. New relationships were built, just as the nurse manager and Dr. Green's had, and other surprising partnerships evolved.

Reflection/Conclusion

After months of preparation and planning, the morning of the move to the new unit finally came. The day began with the physicians walking onto the unit carrying boxes of t-shirts for everyone to wear. The front of the shirts said, "On 4 South, we do it together." The identification of both groups' shared emotions, the interim manager's understanding of emotions and emotion's role in group conflict, her ability to use emotions to reason, and finally, the ability to help the group manage emotions once past the conflict had resolved a serious interdisciplinary conflict. By using EI in collegial relationships, the care teams moved on to new challenges, becoming more effective because of the work they had done.

APPLYING EI ABILITIES TO NURSE TEAM DEVELOPMENT

In addition to using EI abilities to support resolution of interdisciplinary team conflict, EI abilities are also useful in managing professional growth within teams.

Story: The Projector Crisis

The nurse team was a group of experienced, older nurses who had worked together for many years but did not like each other very much. Functional but not inspired, they were at the end stages of their unit's life cycle. Their care was predictable and consistent but not delivered at a very high level of quality. The staff was not interested in professional growth activities and they engaged in education activities reluctantly. There had been recent nursing staff turnover, with the addition of a few younger, more energetic nurses to the team. Their energy and enthusiasm had been greeted with discouraging negativity, and the new cadre was floundering.

The hospital anticipated changes in their client base. The unit's patient population was going to become more acutely ill, and the staff was going to need some new skills. Mandatory retraining was scheduled. Obstacles to success included the staff's resistance to learning and their habit of not working as a team. Changing this would be crucial for success with the new population of patients. Where to begin?

It seemed to the nurse manager that the emotional distance the staff kept from each other prevented them from working as a team. Individual members had many skills and the staff could potentially learn a lot from each other, but the stiff and functional way they interacted and the disinterest with which they regarded each other worked against this. To the nurse manager, the staff seemed like an old couple, sour and grumbly, willing to have dinner together but the rest of the time, sitting in silence at opposite ends of the house.

As she pondered where to begin, the nurse manager was asked by the unit physician group to help them with an international conference they were sponsoring. The conference would attract hundreds of participants and prominent world-class speakers and would be held in a large conference facility. They asked the new manager to take responsibility for the conference, to include conference room organization, media, and introduction of speakers. The manager agreed as long as she got some help. At the next staff meeting, the manager announced to the nursing staff that for the week of the conference, their unit would be closed. The staff would all be required to attend the conference, and their tuition for the event would be paid if they agreed to be on the manager's logistics team. The staff was excited by this plan, which gave them a paid week off work and an exciting new experience.

Applying EI Abilities

Using EI: Identifying Emotions Accurately

At the first staff meeting to discuss the conference, the nurse manager noted the group was energized, a big emotional change from their usual low energy state. Even in day-to-day unit function and bedside patient care, this new group energy was obvious. In Figure 4.1, on the mood and energy graph, the staff as a group had clearly been in Quadrant 1 when the new nurse manager had begun her role in the unit. Overall mood and energy of the unit had been low. Plans for the conference changed this. There was excitement in the air.

Using EI: Understanding Emotions

The nurse manager understood emotional energy is necessary for change. Even negative energy can fuel change, but positive energy goes further and is more constructive. It generates more energy for building relationships, skill development, and learning. As illustrated in Figure 4.1, Mood and Energy Graph, after the announcement of the conference, there was a new energy in the system. The new manager knew this energy could be

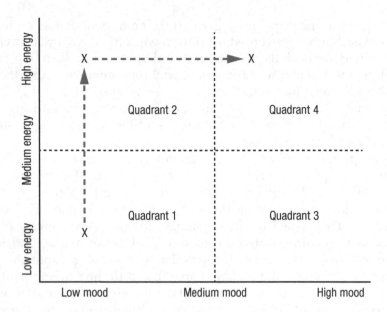

FIGURE 4.1 Graphing team mood and energy.

channeled into improving the emotional climate of the unit and fostering positive change.

Using EI: Using Emotions to Reason

The staff prepared for their support role by reviewing their personalized checklists their manager had made. Each member was assigned a presentation room for a specific time period. The individual assigned to the room was responsible for checking the room setup and media and introducing the speaker at the beginning of each presentation. When their job was completed, the staff was free to roam the conference and enjoy presentations, social events, and conference amenities. As the new responsibilities sunk in, the manager noticed a sense of anxiety among the staff. She knew she was challenging them with a new situation. Many of the older nurses had limited experience with technology and media equipment. Despite practice and reference material several on the staff remained anxious. The manager did not jump to save the nurses from their anxiety. Instead, she waited, a little anxious herself. The new energy in the staff could change the team, and she wanted to see how that might change the group. By understanding anxiety, both hers and the staff's, she reasoned through the situation differently. Anxiety is not always bad. It can be a force for change.

Using EI: Managing Emotions

Shortly before the conference, the group presented her with a revised schedule assigning two people to each conference room. One person was assigned hospitality responsibilities, a strength of the older nurses, and their partner was assigned media and technology responsibilities, a strength of the younger nurses. The partnerships used new relationships to achieve a goal and deal with their anxiety. This solution resulted in less time off at the conference, but greater security in their responsibilities, and more support. The group had decided to work together.

Story Reflection

The day of the conference came, and the manager stopped by the first conference presentation. At the door, one of the older staff members dressed formally in a beautiful suit, warmly welcomed her. Entering the room, she saw a sight that stunned her. The room was large, with over a hundred seats, all empty except for the front row. There, her entire staff sat, shoulder to shoulder, ready to support the two staff assigned to the room if necessary.

The conference changed this team. On the mood/energy graph, the group shifted into Quadrant 4, where energy and mood are both high. The energy generated by the conference and the group's new relationships changed their emotional experience. Mood had lifted. These effects lasted for months after the conference. As a result, clinical care improved. The older staff learned from the recently hired members. When a new care protocol began, bringing with it a challenging patient population and higher acuity, the higher levels of mood and energy helped the staff meet the challenge (see Figure 4.1).

DEVELOPING EMOTIONAL INTELLIGENCE ABILITY

SAMPLE EXERCISE #4: MOOD AND ENERGY MAPPING

In the Mood/Energy story, identification of the unit's mood and energy levels and understanding how mood and energy influence change worked together to support change. The same is true of personal emotional self-management. A self-assessment of emotional mood and overall energy is a way to operationalize the "pulse check" described in a previous chapter. This is easy to do at the beginning of each day. "High mood but low energy: I need to plan an energizing activity before I do anything else!" It is also a great way to begin one-on-one meetings. "Oh! Both of us are low energy.How about we do a walking meeting, to get some energy moving?" Even small groups or classes can benefit from reporting on mood/energy to help plan for the more effective learning/planning.

REFERENCES

Freshwater, D., & Stickley, T. (2004). The heart of the art: Emotional intelligence in nurse education. *Nursing Inquiry, 2*(2), 91–98. https://doi.org/10.1111/J.1440 -1800.2004.00198.x

King, I. (1981). *A theory for nursing: Systems, concepts, process.* Delmar.

Mayer, J. D., Caruso, D., & Salovey, P. (1999). Emotional intelligence meets traditional standards for an intelligence. *Intelligence, 27,* 267–298. https://doi .org/10.1016/S0160-2896(99)00016-1

Peplau, I. (1992). Interpersonal relations: A theoretical framework for application in nursing practice. *Nursing Science Quarterly, 5*(1), 13–18. https://doi.org/10 .1177/089431849200500106

Shanta, L. L., & Connolly, M. (2013). Using King's interacting systems theory to link emotional intelligence and nursing practice. *Journal of Professional Nursing, 29*(3), 174–180. https://doi.org/10.1016/j.profnurs.2012.04.023

5

Emotional Intelligence: Managing Unit Crisis

INTRODUCTION

This chapter uses the four emotional intelligence (EI) abilities, identifying emotions, understanding emotions, using emotions to reason, and managing emotions as a framework for exploring use of EI abilities to manage a unit in crisis (Mayer et al., 1999). Their usual order is adapted to best align with the nursing process. A story illustrates a unit manager's use of EI to manage team dysfunction, problem-solving, and manager self-care.

APPLYING EI ABILITIES TO UNIT CRISIS MANAGEMENT

Story: The Job She Didn't Want

After moving across the country with her new family, the nurse, with an extensive background in nursing management, applied for a critical care staff nurse position. The unit manager position was also open. She didn't want it. The doctors who interviewed her told story after story about patients they had given up on that the staff had pulled through. The nursing staff patiently interviewed her for the staff nurse position she wanted, but their questions kept coming back to her leadership abilities, and her passion for care and development of nurses. Finally, the nurse executive said to her, "Frankly, I have for months been praying that God would send us a healer. I think it is you."

The unit was in trouble, a "fire all the nurses, rehire a new staff and start over" kind of trouble. The nurse executive had been given one last chance before this step would be taken. From the beginning, she had believed this nurse had the skills to help. There was proof that a drug ring was operating out of the unit. Drug theft was ongoing, and the hospital response had been handled badly from the start. Documentation, staff disciplinary action, team intervention, and leadership issues had all been bungled. The staff was traumatized, suspicious, and unsure of whom to trust. Remarkably though, the quality of care on the unit remained high.

As she considered taking the job, the nurse, who had worked with units in trouble before, knew this job had all the earmarks of being the biggest triumph or disaster of her professional life. Later in her life, this story was the one she would always point to, saying, "Without EI, this would have been a disaster." She changed her mind and accepted the position.

During her first staff meeting, the new nurse manager said to the frightened and distraught staff, "I have three things to say to you. First, I have never heard stories like the ones I hear about the exceptional care you give. Second, the crisis this unit faces threatens that care and each of your jobs. Third, I know you guys have gone through hell. We are going to walk out that hell together."

Applying EI Abilities to Management of Leadership Style

Using EI: Identifying, Understanding, and Using Emotions to Reason

This manager had a preferred management style that was collaborative, non-authoritarian, collegial, and heavily focused on professional and personal development and wellness. She and the teams in her care had thrived with this leadership style. Elements of this approach would be needed in the days ahead. The staff was emotionally wounded and traumatized, and at high risk for burnout and emotional trauma. They needed nurturing, healing, and the offering of self-care plans to move forward professionally.

However, progress toward these goals could not be made in an unsafe environment. The ongoing drug diversion created an unsafe situation for caregivers and patients alike. Restoring safety had to be the highest priority. This would require that the nurse manager adopt, at least for a time, a more authoritarian leadership style. Authoritarian leadership is required in "zero error" work (such as nuclear reactors) and in situations where safety has been compromised.

The new nurse manager identified her own emotions related to leadership style and the emotions of her traumatized staff. She understood the emotional implications of various leadership styles on these emotional realities. By identifying and understanding everyone's emotions, she integrated thinking and feeling to consider what kind of leadership was needed.

She managed the staff's emotions by clearly communicating the plan she had for herself, the staff, and the unit. When she first arrived, pervasive fear permeated the unit. This emotion surfaced in nearly every exchange she had with individual staff members about their jobs and the possibility of the unit closing and rehiring new staff, the drug theft everyone knew was going on, and the possibility of being unwittingly associated with the thefts. Some staff were fearful to the point of paralysis. Still others were fearful of their patients' comfort and safety.

The nurse manager understood fear narrows focus and increases perception of threats in the environment. It lowers thresholds for other emotions like frustration and anger. For the staff, frustration and anger would be close to the surface, making relationships more difficult, including her own budding relationships with staff. This identification of fear, combined with an understanding of fear, enabled her to manage emotions in this difficult, emotionally charged situation.

Using EI: Managing Emotions

The manager helped the staff manage their emotions with interventions designed to decrease fear. In staff meetings she gave specific information about what was happening, what she expected of them, and tangible boundaries for their own behavior. The main priority was safety. She was open with the staff, talking about the healing she wanted for them, and the staff development, education, and professional growth she planned for them in the future. She repeated over and over again, "First, we gotta get safe." She used "tough love" and other emotional descriptors to tell them what to expect from her. Her authoritarian style was necessary to make care safe. The staff began to understand this necessity within the context of the crisis their unit faced.

Story Reflection

Leaders typically choose jobs in which their preferred leadership style matches the organization, culture, and staff. But as a practical matter, organizations and work units change continuously. As a unit evolves, it goes through developmental cycles and predictable age cycles. A leadership style that works well in one cycle can be counterproductive in another. A wise and mature leader evolves with their unit and matches their leadership interventions with the needs of the unit. The new manager in this situation chose an initial authoritarian style, with a high degree of structure, accountability, very specific follow-up, and a focus on clear behavioral expectations because her unit needed that kind of leader, for a while.

The nurse manager always valued close relationships with her staff members and worried an authoritarian style, characterized by an emphasis on tangible and specific behavioral outcomes and emotional distance, would inhibit bonding with the staff. However, the staff started to relax.

Their fear and anxiety markedly decreased. Their past mistrust of the administration made had them feel no one was in control. When their new manager stepped up, telling them what to expect and focusing on safety, it communicated, "I got this." The staff quickly began to trust her. They could focus on their work knowing their leader would do what was necessary.

The decrease in fear and anxiety released energy for patient care. A sense of routine returned to the unit. By identifying emotions in the situation, understanding them, using them to reason, and managing them in herself and in a highly emotional situation, the manager normalized unit function and laid groundwork for the hard work ahead.

Applying EI Abilities to Clinical Process Change

With this foundation, the new manager could get into the weeds of the flawed procedures for handling narcotics that put the unit at risk for drug theft. Identification of the individuals stealing drugs would be imperative, but the first priority was to fix the faulty unit processes that made theft possible.

The team's poor narcotic handling processes had set up the unit for drug theft. The team was small and confronting each other was uncomfortable, making changing narcotic handling procedures more difficult. For example, cosigning wastage of narcotic had been accepted as pro forma. When a staff member asked another to cosign the wastage of drug, the cosigning nurse did not insist on observing the actual wastage. This flawed procedure made drug diversion possible. When told to personally observe drug wastage, staff resisted because they did not want to appear to suspect their coworkers. Even on a unit in terrible trouble because of drug diversion, the poor practice of narcotic wastage cosignature was actively supported by the whole staff. When confronted with the need to change this the staff expressed fear of anger and reprisal, as well as fear of compromising friendships among the staff.

Using EI: Identifying, Understanding, Using, and Managing Emotions

Identifying what the staff was feeling was the first step. Understanding the unit's complex psychosocial dynamics helped the new manager think/feel through helping the staff to manage their emotions. She shifted their attention away from their fears about interpersonal challenges. Instead, she helped them emotionally refocus on a more immediate problem than their relationships—the dangers of drug diversion. She repeatedly identified the consequences of not following accurate procedures. She shared her plans to continue tracking "every single milligram" of narcotic moving through the unit. On a clinical unit that had thousands of milligrams of narcotic stored on the unit at any given time, this sounded Herculean! "I don't care if it is only two milligrams you are cosigning! If you cosign it, you are telling me that you vouch for the fact that those two milligrams went in the trash! And that better be true!"

The phrase "every single milligram" came up repeatedly. It was the clarion call to improved performance. Surprisingly quickly, the staff consensus about the importance of this simple but critical process shifted and the practice changed. There was some resistance. Divisions among the staff became obvious. Staff who supported the change and those who did not became obvious, creating group pressure that supported change. Everyone knew whoever was stealing drugs would need to be identified and fired. This, too, caused pressure to support the change in practice. The staff's emotions about their relationships had been blocking the change of practice that was needed. Identifying this, bringing it to the staff's attention, and then helping them refocus on a more serious priority, was key to changing their behavior.

Story Reflection

Complex and serious clinical problems are not solved quickly, but clear, concrete first steps moved this unit one step closer to problem resolution. The drug theft had not been solved nor the guilty parties identified, but the unit was safer because a critical process had been restored. The interpersonal dynamics that put the unit at risk had been confronted and changed. Without the EI abilities described, even this one small first step could have proven difficult. Indeed, the codependent behavior that enabled the drug theft could have made the problem impossible to solve.

Applying EI Ability to Disciplinary Action

Part of the "track every milligram" campaign was to track narcotics from storage through administration and finally to wastage if applicable. If 50 mg were signed out and 25 were given, the documentation in both narcotic tracking and clinical documentation should have totaled 50 mg. Surprisingly, this basic requirement was not being met. Clinical evaluation of pain level and response to pain medication were included in the narcotic tracking. In the nurse manager's initial evaluation of the unit's processes and staff performance, clinical documentation related to pain management did not meet standard practice requirements, another flawed process placing the unit at risk for drug diversion.

The nurse manager summarized the findings from her narcotic handling survey with the staff. She included the total amount of narcotic that could not be accounted for. The data was shocking and made the magnitude of the problem clear: poor drug handling procedures contributed to an environment where it was easy to steal drugs. The manager restated the required standard for narcotic documentation. Every milligram had to be accounted for and reflected in the clinical documentation. Pain level, drug administration, pain relief, and if needed readministration, all had to be documented. She shared her plan to track these requirements and assured the entire staff they would be receiving individual feedback about their performance. No one was singled out.

By this time, the nurse manager had grown close to her staff and had excellent rapport with many of them. These staff members changed their narcotic handling habits quickly as they realized their sloppy practice had contributed to the unit's problem. While monitoring this group's emotional response to the change, the nurse manager identified their emotions and understood their willingness to change behavior reflected an acceptance of responsibility for part of the problem.

Using this "think/feel" process helped the manager plan the next step, using the hospital's formal disciplinary process to confront and document every variation in practice revealed in daily narcotic use surveys. Formal disciplinary meetings were held with every staff member not compliant with required procedures. Human resources documentation of performance expectations was completed and scrupulously followed up on. Tangible expectations with time frames and consequences of failure to improve performance were made clear and documented.

This was the first clear step to identify staff members who were stealing drugs, which the staff had known was coming and feared. Because the investigation was built on a solid foundation of communication and trust, it was surprisingly untraumatic for the staff. For staff who had complied with the process changes and improved their performance, there was no cause for concern. For staff who initially did not improve their performance, a series of disciplinary meetings made them to understand that changing their practice was not optional. These staff were forced into compliance under threat of losing their job. They did not "buy in" to the change, but their behavior changed nonetheless. They complained but got little sympathy. The unit culture had successfully shifted largely as a result of effective use of EI.

Applying EI Ability to Team Dysfunction: Bullying and Codependence

The investigation continued in behind the scenes consultations between the nurse manager and members of the interdisciplinary team, Human Resources, the hospital Employee Assistance program, nursing union representatives, and agents of the local Drug Enforcement Agency. Because

safe procedures for narcotic handling and administration had been restored and the acute phase of staff crisis stabilized, it was time to identify and deal with staff who were diverting drugs. The team had largely
returned to normality. The manager began the individual mentoring and
staff development she had hoped for and the overall morale of the unit
had improved.

However, both the investigation and the disciplinary process had increased pressure on the staff who were stealing drugs. These individuals
were in defensive mode, and the negative behavior that had always characterized their team interactions became more overt. Inappropriate acting
out increased, as did bullying and intimidation. Alarmingly, although the
staff complained, they refused to confront inappropriate behavior, therefore normalizing it and allowing it to continue. As the nurse manager
explored this, identifying the emotional consequences of long-term bullying in the staff, she understood this bullying and resulting codependent
behavior was another risk factor that had set the unit up for the crisis.

Using EI: Identifying Emotions Accurately

Identification of emotions is critical to working with team dysfunction.
Early on, the nurse manager identified a staff culture of codependent behavior. Even when individual staff improved their own drug handling procedures, they struggled to confront other staff members who did not. Even
when working directly with a nurse they believed was diverting narcotics,
they tolerated poor nursing care, inappropriate behavior, and lack of accountability. This long-standing codependent habit only intensified in the
crisis over drug diversion. The nurse manager's identification of the codependence within the staff and her understanding of its role in perpetuating
team dysfunction enabled her to use her emotions to reason that the staff
had to understand their codependence was actively supporting drug theft.

Using EI: Understanding Emotions and Using Them to Reason

Teams do not set out to facilitate unprofessional behavior or put patients
at risk. But when a pattern of behavior within a team has grown into a
habit, the pattern can be hard to break. Bullying works as a habit. Worried about the prospect of confrontation, the staff reverted to fear. After
identifying this and understanding the impact of fear on a change process, the manager chose an educational and behavior change approach.
She drew on what the staff already knew about codependent behavior.
Several had family members in Alcoholics Anonymous and were familiar
with the notion that changing one's behavior is often key to supporting
behavior change in others. Despite this, staff repeatedly expressed fear
and resistance to confronting bullying and inappropriate behavior. Many

were uncomfortable with confrontation and when asked, could not envision how they would go about it.

Using EI: Managing Emotions

Having identified the unit's codependent and bullying emotional habits, applying her understanding of both problems, and after having used both these to think about the situation differently, she made a plan to manage these emotional dysfunctions in the unit. This resulted in a behaviorally focused plan designed to decrease fear and improve confidence. The goal was that this would help the staff confront bullying and change their own codependent behavior. Once a shift, she approached one of the staff who had asked for help in confronting inappropriate behavior. She would do something inappropriate. Throwing something usually worked well. The staff then had to do something, anything! One very shy nurse finally succeeded in responding, "I am very uncomfortable that you did that, and I think you should stop." It became a game. There was nervous laughter, but it got easier. Staff members compared notes about what they would do when the manager threw something next time. With the coaching, peer support, and humor in this approach, the staff confronted inappropriate behavior, breaking their codependence habit.

Story Reflection

Change in staff relationships, patterns of behavior, and the complex social systems by which people in groups work together does not happen easily. For this group of nurses, who had come so far together, this final realization of their own complicity helped them move forward with new skills. The use of EI—identifying emotions, understanding them, using them to reason, and managing them—was key to the nurse manger's success and the unit's healing. The nurse manager and the staff did together, "walk out of hell." Staff who were stealing drugs were identified and fired. The trauma and shame that had hovered over the unit dissipated and was replaced by the staff's pride in the care they gave. The unit's excellent care continued and it became a center for the mentoring of novice nurses.

Applying EI Abilities to Manager Self-Care

Invisible to the staff, the nurse manager had to contend with stress and emotional trauma during the entire process. Self-care throughout the year had been a constant challenge.

Using EI: Identifying Emotions Accurately

Using EI to support self-care begins with the identification of one's emotions. Employing autocratic leadership style left the manager emotionally isolated. In more normal circumstances, relationships with her staff would have been a source of emotional energy and satisfaction. In this case, while emotionally supporting the staff, she could not rely on the team for emotional connection and support. Similarly, the emotional distance required for numerous disciplinary actions contributed to her sense of isolation, fear, self-doubt, and emotional negativity. Her own vulnerability and fear were regular companions as she worked for the unit's healing.

Using EI: Understanding, Using Emotions to Reason, and Managing Emotions

Understanding emotions and how they work was important for her day-to-day well-being. Realizing that emotional isolation can distort emotions, she cultivated a mentor who supported her, several colleagues outside the hospital, and a counselor to help her evaluate her own well-being. The reality checks these relationships provided ensured her emotional problem-solving was not distorted by her own fears and anxieties. Using the think/feel process to reason about her leadership helped her emotionally problem-solve and make plans to manage her own emotional wellness.

NURSING EI RESEARCH, EI AND ENVIRONMENT OF CARE

The earliest EI organizational research provided evidence for the importance of EI in organizations. Nursing research has mirrored the findings of this evidence. There are strong associations between EI and things like team performance, organizational commitment, pro-social behaviors, positive conflict styles, and leadership capabilities (see Chapter 15 for a detailed review of the research).

DEVELOPING EMOTIONAL INTELLIGENCE IN THE CLINICAL ENVIRONMENT

EMOTIONAL INTELLIGENCE DEVELOPMENT SAMPLE EXERCISE #5: TALKING THE WALK

This chapter's story illustrates one of the most important ways to develop EI in teams, talking about plans to address problems. Team emotional problem-solving needs to be openly discussed and specific. The EI abilities can guide this.

1. Identifying emotions: Referring to emotions out loud is a good place to begin. "I am hearing a lot of people sound nervous about ....," or, "I know some of you are angry about ...." Asking about emotions ("How are you feeling about ...?") and referring to them specifically helps the unit be aware of, and accurate with, their emotions both as individuals and as a group.

2. Understanding emotions: Building understanding of emotions should be an ongoing part of staff development. Helping the staff understand codependence, for example, was a critical element for success in this chapter's story. Teaching about emotions as they relate to stress, burnout, change process, and other unit phenomena enhances the staff's emotional capabilities.

3. Using emotions to reason: Teaching staff to think/feel helps the staff deal with conflict, grief, stress, conflict, and other challenges to the unit's emotional health. This is best taught by example, in formal settings like staff meetings or informal change of shift gatherings. "You guys, we have really taken a hit these last few days. We lost a couple of patients we knew well. Our defenses are down. We are hurting and it is an easy time to make mistakes. So, let's take particularly good care of each other today, and be particularly careful with our patients." This comment models good think/feel: identifying the higher than usual risk for error during emotional vulnerability.

4. Emotional problem-solving by managing emotions and emotional situations: Emotional problem-solving needs to be overtly discussed in staff relationships. This can take many forms but begins with managers modeling it in both one-on-one and group interactions. Bering intentional about modeling effective emotional behavior is important. The manager in this story used phrases like, "If I didn't care about you, I wouldn't bother. But I do care about you, so what I need to tell you is ...," It also models being an emotion scientist, using specific language and choosing thoughtful responses over emotional reactivity.

REFERENCE

Mayer, J. D., Caruso, D., & Salovey, P. (1999). Emotional intelligence meets traditional standards for an intelligence. *Intelligence, 27,* 267–298. https://doi.org/10.1016/S0160-2896(99)00016-1

6

Emotional Intelligence in Advanced Practice Nursing

INTRODUCTION

Advanced practice differs from other levels of nursing in depth, scope, and role, and emotional intelligence (EI) abilities are one means by which these differences can be developed. This chapter illustrates the four EI abilities: identifying emotions, understanding them, using emotions to reason, and emotional management as they apply to advance practice nursing (Mayer et al., 1999). Their usual order is adapted to best align with the nursing process.

APPLYING EI TO ADVANCED NURSING PRACTICE

Story: Once Upon a Canoe, a Transcript

The nurse practitioner was called to see a newly diagnosed diabetic refusing treatment. A late middle-aged man with no family, the patient appeared well dressed, intelligent, shy, and determined to refuse treatment for his diabetes. When asked why, he shrugged and said, "No point." His nurses made repeated attempts to do diabetes education, all unsuccessful, so they had called the hospital APRN diabetes nurse for help. The APRN entered his room, sat, and introduced herself. The patient was polite, but answered her questions with short, single-word answers.

> APRN: So I see that you are not retired. What is your occupation?
> Patient: I was a wilderness guide in the outback of Canada.
> APRN: So, canoes then?
> Patient: Yes.
> APRN: What make of canoe?
> Patient: (hesitates) Grumman's.
> APRN: So, you know that small thwart behind the back seat? The little one?

Patient nods but does not say anything, looking puzzled.

APRN: That is where you'll need to lash your diabetes kit.

Patient makes eye contact for the first time, but continues to look puzzled.

APRN: Because we both know sooner or later you are going to swamp, at least partially if the water gets bad, so you want to make sure your kit is attached right to the canoe. Even if it goes over, your kit will stay put.

Patient: What?

APRN: You will have to be really careful to make sure your kit is totally safe, right?

Patient: I can't do that.

APRN: You can't do what?

Patient: I can't be a diabetic and an outback guide.

APRN: Well, you can of course choose not to be a guide anymore if you want, but there is no reason why you can't manage your diabetes just fine while you are in the outback. You will need to plan food a bit differently and get good at watching your blood sugar levels, but hey, it is just one more part of the trip, right?

Patient looks surprised, but picks up one of the teaching pamphlets.

APRN: So, if you are okay with this, let's talk about a few basics about having diabetes.

Applying EI Abilities

APRNs are experts in their profession. The APRN in this story did an assessment of this patient that was subtle, deep, and fast. Experts in practice deal with a situation as a whole, without relying on the accumulation of many facts before understanding a situation. This can result in a rapid perception of a gestalt, a totality of a situation often described as intuitive, but is actually an advanced form of perception and analysis characteristic of the expert practitioner at this level. There is little research on this phenomenon, but it is possible that EI abilities facilitate this rapid perception, analysis, and problem-solving.

This APRN did not take a whole interview to understand what was going on with this patient. In a short period of time, this APRN got past the patient's misunderstanding, past his defenses, and by aligning with his priorities, got to the heart of the matter. The interaction took no more than 10 minutes. That the APRN was familiar with canoes helped, but it was her astute EI ability that facilitated her breakthrough. Table 6.1 illustrates the use of the four EI abilities across the interaction between the nurse and patient. The APRN's rapid thinking and insight were certainly not in the full thoughts and sentences explicated in the table description. These descriptions, rather, flesh out the way the EI abilities were being used in the interaction.

TABLE 6.1 Once Upon a Canoe: Dialogue Analysis EI Abilities

DIALOGUE	INTEGRATION OF EI ABILITY
APRN: I see that you are not retired. What is your occupation? Patient: "I was a wilderness guide in the outback of Canada." *EI Ability: Identifying emotions*	The APRN noticed the patient referred to himself in the past tense. He was not retired and had no family. His job as an outback guide was likely the core reality of his life, his identity. This man's grief was so profound that he was referring to himself in the past tense.
APRN: So, canoes then? Patient: Yes. APRN: What make? Patient: (hesitates) Grumman's. APRN: The new ones? Patient: (hesitates) No, I like the old heavy ones. They stand up better. *EI Ability: Understanding emotions*	The assumption that having diabetes meant he lost his identity had several implications: (1) He was grieving a loss. (2) False thinking led to false perception. (3) He could draw on his capability and passion in canoeing to manage his diabetes. Understanding this constellation of false thinking, grief, and despair, she could think differently.
APRN: So, you know that small thwart behind the back seat? The little one? That is where you'll need to lash your insulin kit. Patient: (Making eye contact but continues to look puzzled.) APRN: Because we both know sooner or later you are going to swamp, at least partially if the water gets bad, so you want to make sure your kit is attached right to the canoe. Even if it goes over, your kit will stay put. Patient: What? APRN: You will have to be really careful to make sure your kit is totally safe. Patient: I can't do that. APRN: You can't do what? Patient: I can't be a diabetic and an outback guide. *EI Ability: Understanding and managing emotions*	Think/feeling helped the APRN realize that (1) inaccurate thinking created maladaptive behavior, and (2) she needed to break through this false thinking. To do this she used her knowledge of canoes to assist him in shifting his thinking about himself, diabetes, and his life as a guide. By doing this, the APRN challenged his false thinking. In response the patient was able to say out loud the false thing he had been thinking.

(continued)

TABLE 6.1 Once Upon a Canoe: Dialogue Analysis EI Abilities (*Continued*)

DIALOGUE	INTEGRATION OF EI ABILITY
APRN: (Pauses a minute). Well, you can of course choose not to be a guide anymore if you want, but there is no reason why you can't manage your diabetes just fine while you are guiding. You will need to plan food a bit differently and get good at watching your blood sugar levels, but hey, it is just one more part of the trip, right? *EI Ability:* Managing emotions	The APRN knew that until the patient had confronted his false thinking, he would not be able to replace it with new information. Once the patient had spoken the false thinking out loud, it was time to offer new, accurate information. In these few words, she also invited him back into the world he thought he had lost, with a challenge to deal with, certainly, but a doable challenge.
Patient: (Looks surprised, but picked up one of the teaching pamphlets.) APRN: So, if you are okay with this, let's talk about a few basics about having diabetes. *EI Abilities:* Identifying, Understanding, Using, and Managing emotions	This APRN knew that learning can be blocked by emotions. The emotional processes of grief and loss were completely blocking this patient's ability to accept being a diabetic. With his false ideas about diabetes, he could not combine the "outback guide" part of his self-concept with "diabetic." Once he began to be able to do this, he began to be open to learning about diabetes. The way that the APRN focused on canoes, not diabetes, was an effective way of helping the patient shift his false thinking to a beginning for being able to accept diabetes treatment.

APPLYING EI ABILITIES TO ADVANCED PRACTICE TEACHING

Story: The Heart of 911

September 11, 2001, the clinical nurse specialist (CNS) nurse educator came to work early to set up for a day-long cardiac pathophysiology class. It was a mandatory session for a group of nurses at the end of a critical course, right before the final exam. As she organized the classroom, a member of the housekeeping staff arrived to assist. He did not pick up chairs or move tables. He just looked at her with a stunned look on his face and he told her about the first plane that had hit the tower in New York City, and about the second one. "My cousin works in that area," he said.

That day would be a turning point in history, but that morning, the instructor had a room full of nurses to teach. The class could not be cancelled or postponed. It was one of the most important and most difficult classes in the course and the final exam was only days away. But even in her own shock and distress, she knew that she had to find a way to help her students get through the day. Learning was a priority, but many of the students were spouses of military personnel stationed in the area. Some had family in New York. Others had family members traveling, now stranded as airports closed. There was also emotional work to be done. How could she teach cardiac physiology on a day like this?

The CNS started the class and encouraged them to talk about the events of the morning. Then she shared the revised plan for the day. They would still cover course material to prepare for the exam, but class breaks would be longer, and the televised news would be set up in the break room. The class format, however, would change. The instructor would use the same PowerPoint presentation about normal anatomy and physiology of the heart and material about a wide range of pathologies, but she wanted to change the layout of the room. With the students' help, she moved the large classroom chairs out of their usual rows and used them as building blocks to construct the outline of a huge heart. The outline included the great vessels leading to and from the heart, and an area labeled "lungs." Inside the outline of the heart were its internal chambers and valves.

The nurse educator handed each class member a blue balloon to symbolize a deoxygenated hemoglobin cell. Each student entered the heart through one of the great vessels, walked through the valves and chambers of the heart and ended up in the lungs, where they exchanged their blue balloon for a red one, representing an oxygenated hemoglobin cell. As the group walked through the heart repeatedly, they discussed normal functioning of the heart, its normal pressures, cycles, sounds, and phenomena. The students giggled as "atrial kick" pushed them out of the atria through a valve and into a ventricle. The energy of the class rose and people began to relax.

Over the day, disease by disease, the "chair-built heart" was modified to represent a wide range of diseases. The CNS would ask, "How would aortic stenosis change the normal heart?" and the students would adjust the chairs depicting the aorta, narrowing the passageway. Then the class would walk through the heart with their balloons. Questions came up along the way. "Okay, you guys in the aorta, what is going on?" Students answered, "We can't get through. It is too tight!" She would pose, "Okay, so what is happening with you guys in the ventricle?," and students would respond, "Things are backing up. It is getting congested in here! The pressure is rising!"

PowerPoint slides covering each pathology were projected on the wall. The class walked through the heart repeatedly, creating and experiencing pathological change represented by each of the diseases. They answered questions describing the ways normal function, pressures, structures, and cardiac phenomena like oxygen consumption changed with each pathology. The class took frequent breaks and shared stories and family concerns. When they returned to class, they picked up their balloons and walked through the heart again.

Applying EI Abilities in Teaching

This CNS nurse educator used EI abilities in very simple and tangible ways to create effective learning despite the emotional obstacles of that day. She used the learning activity as emotional medicine to care for shocked and traumatized students. This CNS not only taught difficult course content but on the fly, totally changed the class presentation so the class could learn effectively in an extreme emotional circumstance that could have prevented learning. The nurse educator did these things simultaneously, with no preparation and little time, amid a moment of history in which she too, had family and friends at risk, exemplifying advance practice nursing. How was she able to do this? The case can be described in terms of EI abilities. Like many nurses who use EI abilities, she was not consciously using them, but she was using them nonetheless.

Using EI: Identifying Emotions

The nurse educator began by identifying emotions, beginning with her own. Considering her huge challenge ahead, she wanted to be both teacher and healer. Her own feelings could have made it difficult to be either. Even though time was short, she dedicated a few minutes to calling her own family. Once the class arrived, the instructor addressed the shock, fear, pain, and anxiety she knew they all were feeling. That so many of the class members had spouses in the military added uncertainty about the future into the mix. As the group shared their worry, unexpected concerns like possible deployment or relocation were added to the list of emotions the group members shared. Identifying these feelings out loud was a first step for the challenging emotional problem-solving that lay ahead. In addition to the emotions from the events of the day, the nurses also talked about anxiety related to the class itself. They had already been anxious about the course content for the day. Most of the class was uncomfortable with cardiac pathophysiology. Many in the class had done poorly on the course pretest cardiac disease questions and were anxious about the final exam.

Using EI: Understanding Emotions

As an advance practice nurse teacher, the educator was an expert on the relationship between emotions and learning. She understood that shock is a powerful protective emotion that can negatively affect learning and that physiologically, the fight/flight mechanism reduces ability to focus enough to take in new information. The fight/flight emotions (the fear, anxiety, anger, and frustration felt by group) could impair their ability to take in new information and learn. As healer/teacher, her efforts to

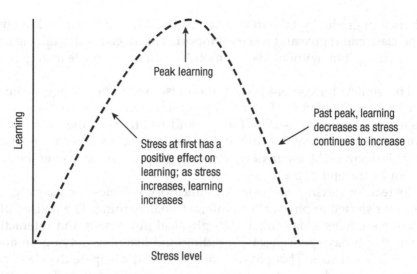

FIGURE 6.1 Stress curve and learning.

teach might not only be ineffective but could increase anxiety unless the powerful emotions from that morning were addressed. She also understood about the anxiety curve and learning; increased anxiety initially enhances the focus and attention needed for learning, but past a certain point, anxiety inhibits learning (see Figure 6.1).

Using EI: Using Emotions to Reason

Having identified and understood the powerful emotions in her class, the APRN used these two EI abilities to reason. Characteristic of advance practice, this process was subtle, deep, and fast and she managed the situation as a complex and dynamic whole. She did not have time for detailed analysis, fact finding, or the individual assessment of each class member to decide the best approach. In this complex and dynamic "think/feel" process, emotions informed reasoning and reasoning informed emotional processes. This laid a solid foundation for the emotional problem-solving necessary to plan.

Using EI: Managing Emotions in Oneself and in Emotional Situations

Beginning the class with talking about what had happened gave the nurses time to share their feelings. Class members who had family in New York, spouses deployed near the city, or family in airports shared their concerns. This created individual and group support. During class breaks, students had the chance to call family and friends or watch breaking news on TV. This helped address their shock and gave them a chance to gradually take in and accept what had happened. Members of the class could give and receive support. This decreased available time for teaching, but without basic emotional support, no learning could occur.

The vehicle for content presentation also had to be changed. The instructor kept the planned PowerPoint presentation as part of the class. It was a familiar and reassuring format, and printouts of the presentation gave the students a way to study if they could not yet focus on class material. This decreased their anxiety, reducing the pressure to master the class content by the end of the day.

Instead of relying on visual and auditory vehicles for learning, the instructor shifted to physical and interactional learning. The revised plan gave the students a day filled with physical movement and interaction rather than a day spent passively sitting and listening, relying on auditory and visual cues. This physical outlet helped dissipate the class' fear and anxiety, which raised sympathetic nervous stimulation. The effect of this on large muscles is to make a person want to move! This emotional positivity and physicality gave the class a physical outlet and made it easier to focus on the course material being presented. Offering the class members breaks to watch the news coverage or be in touch with family members helped reduce anxiety and fear.

Story Reflection

The CNS used EI abilities to enable learning and support her class amid emotional trauma. The class learned effectively and experienced emotional healing. When the nurses left the class that day, they had learned, but also had begun healing. They could go back to their families and friends ready to work together to deal with 9/11. The instructor, as an advance practice expert, was able to pull all this off on the fly, with no preparation and no advance planning.

RESEARCH FINDINGS: APPLICATION OF EI TO ADVANCED PRACTICE

Beyond the large body of research on nurse leader EI, very little research exists specific to EI in advanced practice nursing. However, the nursing leadership EI research findings likely apply to other advanced practice roles. The core competencies that overlap among these roles are associated with EI ability, such as interpersonal effectiveness, organizational adaptation, teamwork, stress resilience, and long-term thriving (see Chapter 15 for a detailed review of this research). In one conceptual analysis of the relationship between EI abilities, APRN competencies and Quality and Safety Education for Nurses (QSEN) Competencies, EI competencies consistently corresponded with important APRN outcomes (Cox, 2018).

EMOTIONAL EDUCATION IN ADVANCED PRACTICE NURSING

Education for advance practice nursing is outlined in the *Essentials of Master's Education in Nursing* (American Association of Colleges of Nursing [AACN], 2011). There are nine "essentials"that outline the knowledge and skill acquisition required of APRNs.

The curriculum outlined in *Essentials*

1. Core content for masters' students in the four APRN roles.
2. Patient care core competencies relevant to patient care given at an advanced level.
3. Functional content appropriate for each of the advanced practice roles.

The nine competencies address capabilities required to operationalize these three main categories of competency (see Table 6.2). In addition to these requirements, APRN's are expected to lead, act as change agents, advance lifelong learning and cultures of excellence, build and lead collaborative interprofessional teams, expertly navigate and integrate health care services across the healthcare system, and innovate and translate research evidence into practice (AACN, 2011).

The *Essentials of Master's Education in Nursing* does not address the emotional abilities required for masters' preparation. To illustrate this, each of the nine core essentials was reviewed to identify possible association with EI competencies. Only once in the entire document was the word "emotion" used across all the goals and sample content attached to each of the nine essentials ("Emotional needs," Essential VII). Only six of the Essentials referenced communication skills in an interpersonal context. Reviewing desired outcomes for APRN's across all nine essentials, every one of them is predicated on good communication, effective interpersonal relationships, both formal and informal leadership ability, and the ability to initiate, support, and sustain systems change, all of which depend on EI abilities. Because the essentials document outlines knowledge and skills that all APRN's must master, the absence of reference to emotional capabilities indicates a deficit in graduate education for nurses. Because EI theory operationalizes emotional abilities that are the foundation of effective communication, interpersonal, and team relationships, use of EI abilities in the Essentials document could contribute significantly to APRN education (Table 6.2).

TABLE 6.2 Analysis of Essentials Nursing Practice: References to Emotional Content

ESSENTIAL ITEM	IDENTIFIED CONTENT FIELDS THAT INFORM THE ESSENTIAL	REFERENCES TO EMOTIONS IN DOCUMENT
Essential I: Background for Practice from Sciences and Humanities	Biopsychosocial fields, genetics, public health, quality improvement, organizational sciences	Health communication, Biopsychosocial fields (practice grounded in)
Essential II: Organizational and Systems Leadership	Organizational and systems leadership, ethics, critical decision-making, performance measures, application of quality improvement principles	"effective working relationships," "respectful communication," Communication as an essential skill, and "Effective communication"
Essential III: Quality and Safety	Methods, tools performance standards that relate to quality, quality principles within organizations	"High-level communication skills"
Essential IV: Translating and Integrating Scholarship	Application of research outcomes in practice, resolving practice problems, change agency, dissemination of research	None
Essential V: Informatics and Healthcare Technologies	Use of technology to enhance care and as a communication tool to integrate and coordinate care	"communication technologies"
Essential VI: Health Policy and Advocacy	Intervention in policy process, advocacy strategies	None
Essential VII: Interprofessional Collaboration	Communication, collaboration, consultation with interprofessional teams to manage and coordinate care	Communication, "Multiple intelligences," and "Emotional needs"
Essential VIII: Population Health	Organizational, client-centered, culturally appropriate, clinical prevention and population-based care	None

(continued)

TABLE 6.2 Analysis of Essentials Nursing Practice: References to Emotional Content (*Continued*)

ESSENTIAL ITEM	IDENTIFIED CONTENT FIELDS THAT INFORM THE ESSENTIAL	REFERENCES TO EMOTIONS IN DOCUMENT
Essential IX: Master's-Level Nursing Practice	Science base to master's level practice, supporting direct and indirect care of patients, families and populations	Communication

Source: American Association of Colleges of Nursing. (2011). *The essentials of master's education in nursing*. (p. 4–5). https://www.tnecampus.org/sites/default/files/docs_and_pdfs/Masters%20Essentials.pdf

DEVELOPING EMOTIONAL INTELLIGENCE

SAMPLE EMOTIONAL INTELLIGENCE DEVELOPMENT EXERCISE #6: BRAIN DRAIN

One teacher, at the beginning of each class, led the class in an exercise called "Brain Drain." To do this exercise, students took out a blank sheet of paper and when a bell rang, started writing. There was only one rule: start writing and don't stop for three minutes. They could write anything they wanted to, but they were encouraged to "empty their emotional pockets" before class began. At the end of class, everyone ripped their pieces of paper to shreds and dropped them in the trash can the teacher carried around the room for them. The idea was, get it all out so you can focus on class.

Advanced practice nurses, no matter the role they are in, and no matter the clinical practice area, have one role challenge in common. They are beset, all day, every day, with one challenge after the next, one problem after the next. The next patient appears before the NP is emotionally done with the last one. The emotions of the day, as a leader, a teacher, or a bedside practitioner, pile one upon the next. By the end of the day, it is easy for this emotional backlog to contribute to compassion fatigue and decreased resilience. The Brain Drain exercise is a good one for day's end, just for 3 minutes. After a particularly intense emotional experience, doing a brain drain in the middle of the day might also be useful!

REFERENCES

American Association of Colleges of Nursing. (2011). *The essentials of masters' education in nursing.* https://www.tnecampus.org/sites/default/files/docs _and_pdfs/Masters%20Essentials.pdf

Cox, K. M. (2018). Use of emotional intelligence to enhance advanced practice registered nurse competencies. *Journal of Nursing Education, 57*(11), 648–654. https://doi.org/10.3928/01484834-20181022-04

Mayer, J. D., Caruso, D., & Salovey, P. (1999). Emotional intelligence meets traditional standards for an intelligence. *Intelligence, 27,* 267–298. https://doi .org/10.1016/S0160-2896(99)00016-1

7

Emotional Intelligence in Critical Care Nursing

INTRODUCTION

Emotional intelligence (EI) is defined as the "ability to recognize the meanings of emotions .... and to reason and problem-solve on the basis of them" (Mayer et al., 1999, p. 267). In this chapter, EI is operationally defined with the following abilities:

1. Accurate identification of emotions in self and others
*2. Understanding emotions
*3. Using emotions to reason (integrating thinking and feeling)
4. Managing emotions.
(Mayer et al., 1999).

For the purposes of this text, skills 2 and 3 are reversed from the published Mayer et al. (1999) order. This better aligns the EI abilities with the nursing process illustrated throughout this chapter

Emotional, interpersonal, and social abilities are often referred to as "soft skills." When compared with typical ICU nurse skills, like CPR, hemodialysis, cardiac monitoring, and complex burn wound care, emotional abilities seem "soft" indeed. However, these "soft" skills have an enormous impact on how, when, where, and why technical skills are used. Fear of breaking a rib can inhibit effective CPR. In an interdisciplinary team, defensiveness can impair an effective plan of care. Lack of trust may keep a family from supporting good end-of-life choices for their family member. Unidentified nurse burnout can result in missed assessment cues, slow emergency response, and impaired performance, threatening patient safety. Without "soft skills," care may be at best ineffective and at worst harmful to the patient, their loved ones, and the care team. Given the importance of emotional intelligence (EI) abilities for patient care, team effectiveness, and nurse survival, they can be considered core competencies for critical care nursing.

Story: Uncomfortable But True

The physician examined the patient, who, after days of crisis, was finally stable. After washing her hands, the doctor paused briefly at the door to make eye contact with the nurse for the first time. "When you take care of my patients, they get better," she said before leaving.

After the first blush of the compliment, the nurse was taken aback and a little offended. "We are all great nurses here," she told herself.

As soon as the words left her mouth, she realized this is a common misconception. Nurses are not all the same. Patient outcomes are related to nursing competency, and competency varies. This is nowhere in nursing more obvious than in critical care nursing, where consistency, speed, and accuracy of performance saves lives. Understanding this performance variation among critical care nurses is important.

APPLYING EI TO CRITICAL CARE NURSE PERFORMANCE

Performance and EI Ability

Some critical care nurses perform better than other nurses and their patients have better clinical outcomes. These star performers also avoid burnout and thrive and deepen in professional wisdom across long careers. How are they different? Personality, values, professionalism, education, mentoring, and culture are all factors. Also, EI abilities, which correlate with both performance and professional thriving. The significance of this for critical care nurses is enormous. The impact of EI abilities on critical care nurse performance is easy to recognize, particularly in physiological crisis assessment, acute clinical decision-making and crisis response.

Applying EI Abilities to Clinical Assessment

Using EI: Identifying Emotions

Acute and highly sensitive assessment skills, particularly those that identify imminent life-threatening physiological changes, are among the most important for critical care nurses. Recognition of very subtle changes that presage physiological deterioration enables initiation of treatment before a crisis progresses. One of these first signs of imminent physiological deterioration is an affective, emotional change in the patient. How many times have great nurses said, "My patient just doesn't look right," or "He just isn't himself today," and increased their frequency and depth of follow-up assessment, averting an impending physiological crisis?

Expression of personality and emotional affect require energy. If a patient is in the very early stages of physiological deterioration, they may not have the energy these require. If a nurse accurately identifies premonitory emotions, they may be particularly alert to other, later signs acute of physiological deterioration. In this case, accurate identification of emotions is lifesaving.

Using EI: Understanding Emotions

Paramedics arrive at the home of a person with chest pain and begin their assessment of the patient. The presentation is ambiguous, and the paramedics are unsure if the patient should be transported to the hospital. The patient says, "I am sure it is nothing. I will be fine. You can leave now."

Immediately, the paramedics transport the patient to the hospital. This is not because paramedics are perverse. Rather, they recognize denial as one of the symptoms of a deteriorating cardiac condition. This is an example of acute clinical assessment in which emotions play a critical role. Premonitions of death or crisis are another example. Many patients in early stages of acute physiological deterioration say things like, "Something is wrong," or, "I don't feel right." Understanding this, experienced critical care nurses include these in clinical assessment. Again, this combination of identification of emotions and understanding their significance can be lifesaving.

Applying EI to Clinical Decision-Making

Story: Nurse Anxiety and Titration of Vasoactive Medications

In one ICU that I worked, many of our patients were on continuous intravenous drip medications for blood pressure control. Titrating dosage of these vasoactive medications, which have many potentially harmful side effects, was among the most challenging parts of my work. As a novice in the unit, I observed closely how experienced nurses accomplished this critically important goal. Some nurses were better at this than others. Why? As I asked questions and learned as much as I could about pharmacology, physiology, and other variables that affect drug weaning, I realized something else was involved: nurses' emotions. Even with this seemingly very technical skill, experienced nurses integrated what they knew with how they felt. This affected their patient's clinical outcomes.

Applying EI Abilities

Using EI: Identification of Emotions

This is easily illustrated in the simple steps involved in vasoactive drug weaning. This process begins with observing baseline blood pressure, making a very small change in the intravenous medication rate and observing the patient's response. If the blood pressure remains unchanged, later, another small change can be made, observation of blood pressure stability continued and hopefully this process is repeated over time until the patient is successfully weaned off the medication. What can happen, however, is that a small change is made, and the patient, who has gotten used to depending on the medication, has a drop in blood pressure. At this point, some anxious nurses returned the medication back up to the original dose, or, if the nurse was very anxious, an even higher dose. If the blood pressure went too high as a result, the nurse's anxiousness increased, and she would rapidly turn the medication down, putting the patient on a blood pressure roller coaster. In this case, poorly managed nurse anxiety resulted in physiological instability.

Using EI: Understanding, Using, and Managing Emotions

My mentor did this very differently. She would make a small decrease in medication dose, and, at the bedside together, we would watch the blood pressure drop. I myself got anxious! My mentor would say, "I know this is nerve-racking, but let's take a breath and see if the patient can adapt to this lower dose. Sometimes it takes a few minutes." At the bedside, we would watch as the blood pressure stayed low for a few minutes, then gradually return to baseline. Homeostasis was restored. While continuing to observe the blood pressure carefully, we would wait for a while and repeat the procedure. Not only was this often successful, but it also resulted in fewer "roller coasters" of high and low swings in blood pressure that can result in more instability. A good patient outcome meant paying attention to, and managing, my own anxiety.

Story Reflection

Over time, I noticed that the best nurses, cognizant of drug side effects, always made weaning these medications a high priority. Other nurses did not. I believed the difference lay in the nurses' ability to manage their own anxiety. Avoiding anxiety, usually unconsciously, can mean avoiding the weaning process altogether. The negative clinical outcome is more time on the drugs, a greater chance of side effects, longer ICU stays, and longer hospitalizations. Failure to identify an emotion, to understand it, and "think/feel" through it, directly affects patient outcomes.

Applying EI Abilities in Crisis Management

Managing cardiac arrest and acute resuscitation events require a nurse to assess and intervene astutely and rapidly. The stakes could not be higher. To perform well, critical care nurses must know about drugs, protocols, equipment, and cardiac dysrhythmia. They must be able to do CPR, cardiac monitoring, defibrillation, and management of cardiac pacemakers. But those two categories, things to know and things to do, are not enough for a successful resuscitation. Critical care nurses must also manage the resuscitation process itself, guiding team members and families through the event. Code teams that work well together perform better in codes and their patients have better clinical outcomes.

Using EI: Identifying Emotions

A nurse who identifies their own emotions, understands them, and uses them to reason, can manage them more effectively. This is particularly important in crisis response. For example, if a nurse finds her patient not breathing, the normal psychological response to this traumatic situation is shock and denial. "Oh No! This can't be happening!". A nurse with EI abilities can quickly say, "This is shock and denial. What do I understand about these feelings? They often come up in situations like this, but now I have to take action." This nurse identifies the emotions, understands them, and thinks with them. These emotions do not keep the nurse from taking action. This happens in a split second. The nurse takes a deep breath and takes action.

What if this is not the case? When shock and denial are not identified, their paralytic effect can blunt perception and prevent the rapid actions that are needed. Instead of immediately assessing the patient and pushing the code button, this nurse might call for help or ask that another nurse validate their assessment. In that case, not using EI ability wastes precious, life-saving minutes.

Using EI: Understanding, Using, and Managing Emotions

As the resuscitative effort continues, EI abilities help critical care staff save energy, focus attention, and prioritize, especially while self-managing the adrenalin dump that accompanies every code. Code team members are under the influence of fight/flight neurochemicals. This affects them physically. Their large, adrenalin-fueled muscles predispose them to physically move too much during the code. A common example is the nurse who runs to get equipment from a storage room instead of taking it off the code card. They may talk too much and too loudly and not listen. These behaviors are common in codes. They disrupt resuscitative efforts, waste time, and result in increased error and patient risk. A critical care nurse with good EI skills can identify adrenalin-fueled emotions, understand their effects, use them to reason, and self-manage themselves. This nurse is calm, quiet, focused, listening carefully, and staying still, all of which contribute to better patient outcomes.

APPLYING EI ABILITIES TO RELATIONSHIPS WITH COLLEAGUES AND TEAMS

EI Abilities Applied

Research findings reveal that EI abilities keep communication, relationships, and teamwork effective and healthy. This is important because critical care nursing is a team endeavor, requiring interpersonal support and good teamwork. Good communication is essential. Patients in this setting are unstable and in both psychological and physiological danger. Caring for them is physically, mentally, emotionally, and spiritually challenging. Many elements of this setting challenge good communication. Critical care units are noisy, visually distracting, emotionally distressing, and constantly changing. The emotional environment regularly includes pain, suffering, trauma, and death. These elements can compromise the quality and effectiveness of the communication required for patient care and safe and effective unit function. Maintaining good communication in this setting is not only essential for patient care, but for the interpersonal and team relationships that keep patients safer, foster less turnover, and prevent burnout. This not only improves clinical outcomes but also preserves the reservoir of clinical wisdom that long-serving nurses accumulate.

Because of the intrinsic high level of stress in critical care environments, interpersonal and team relationships are perpetually at risk for miscommunication from misunderstandings or unresolved conflict. Miscommunication slows teamwork and increases error risk. In very busy units, when such interpersonal bumps occur, they can easily get buried by the next crisis of the day. If the conflict is left unaddressed, it can fester and affects both those involved as well as their team. This can distract everyone, sap energy, increase distraction, and compound the miscommunication. In a clinical crisis, this can prevent staff from functioning quickly and effectively.

Story: I Have a Bone to Pick With You!

One unit had an effective, easy way of managing this common problem. They used two simple phrases to manage conflict. The first was, "I have a bone to pick with you." This was an easy way to say, "Something happened between us. I can't get past it and I need your help." Another phrase was, "We need to get the air clear," to indicate something had occurred that was hanging in the air, distracting and sapping energy. These phrases indicated good intent and carried no blame or judgment.

Using EI: Identifying, Understanding, Using, and Managing Emotions

Both these phrases were a function of EI ability. They required nurses to identify negative, conflict-related emotions. ("I am still mad about what happened on the way to the operating room.") They necessitated understanding of the emotion's possible negative effects for patient care and team function. ("If I don't clear the air, working together will be hard, and our care might suffer.") The staff had to use their emotions to reason about the problem. ("I can't shake this feeling, so it needs to be confronted. Then we can get back to working together well.") Lastly, they had to emotionally problem-solve to manage emotions to prevent compromise in team performance.

EI APPLIED TO BURNOUT AND SALUTOGENESIS

EI abilities can be used for burnout prevention, healing, and long-term professional thriving. The general nursing literature (see Chapter 15) provides evidence that greater EI ability correlates with less burnout, less perceived stress, and both physical and emotional wellness. Although there is not yet a substantive corresponding body of evidence for critical care nurses, the same correlations may exist. Further, the salutogenic (wellness generating) effects of EI ability may well contribute to long term healing and thriving of critical care nurses. This is related to two effects of EI abilities. The first is their healing effect on emotional trauma. The second is their positive effect on emotional resilience.

Story: Burned in Half (A Flashback)

A flashback brought it all back many years later. As she revisited the memory, time and time again, all she could see was the same blank wall. With a pounding heart and oppressive fear, she tried to see more. What was in front of that blank wall? She kept trying to see what she was not seeing. What had been there that was too painful, too frightening, even years later, to see? What was she blocking?

Finally, she recognized the image, a blank wall in the trauma resuscitation unit, near the helicopter landing pad. With that revelation, she could see and hear what she had blocked out, what was in front of the wall, and what she had seen and heard and felt that terrible day. She could finally cry. She could finally speak the story out loud.

She had been a good nurse that day, doing what needed to be done. She moved quickly, thought on her feet, worked with the team. They had not been able to save that woman, burned into pieces, with her last breath screaming for her baby. But they had saved others across that long day. She did not remember them, but the baby and the mother stayed hidden, no tears shed, for many years. Until now.

Story: I Love You

She had taken care of a young man with an overwhelming lung disease for months. The entire time she had known him, he had been on a ventilator, making it impossible for him to speak. In the primary care nursing unit, she had cared for him every day. She had seen him through crashes and slow painstaking improvement. She had seen him desperate, psychotic, delirious out of his mind, quiet, peaceful.

She had tried to play gin rummy with him one day, despite the tubes and intravenous lines in every extremity and on a ventilator. She had never seen a patient on a ventilator try to laugh like he did during that game. Returning to work after a vacation, she heard in a report that he was stable and off the ventilator. She walked to his room and leaned on the door jam, watching him, his face finally happy and quiet. She caught his eye and threw her arms in the air, and exclaimed, unashamed tears of joy running down her face, "Talk to me, say something, say anything, recite the alphabet. I have to hear your voice!"

He met her eyes, cleared his throat, and said, "I love you."

Story Reflections: The Salutogenic Effect of EI Ability

The emotional labor of working in critical care environments is multifaceted and incalculable. Stress is in the DNA of these units, it is intrinsic. The physical, cognitive, and emotional labor required constantly challenges nurses' bio-psycho-spiritual wellness. Burnout prevention and wellness sustenance must be serious business for nurses, for both short-term thriving and long-term career wellness. The two previous stories represent two poles of this work, healing and salutogenesis.

Critical care nurses constantly witness acute and chronic crises in patients' lives. What nurses see, hear, smell, and experience create both acute and chronic stress, leading to physical and emotional unwellness. The first story illustrates some elements of this. Critical care nurses must develop not just defensive emotional capabilities and burnout prevention, but also abilities that help them process what they have seen, felt, and remembered. The emotional work necessary to heal flashbacks and traumatic memories may be improved with accurate identification, understanding, think/feeling, and managing of emotions. This use of EI for healing the wounds of emotional labor is one pole of self-care for critical care nurses.

The second story represents the other pole, which is salutogenic, wellness and resilience generating. Despite the emotional labor of her relationship with her patient, the nurse had a salutogenic relationship with him; one that generated wellness, strength, and capability in the nurse. Her love and care for the patient, and his love for her, made her stronger and wiser. The experience of caring for him, the joy and success of his healing, promoted her own wellness and capability.

This salutogenic mutuality is an aspect of the therapeutic relationship that is particularly important within the intimacy and intensity of relationships critical care nurses often develop with their patients. This depth of relationship improves clinical outcomes. Many critical care nurses are aware of this in emotionally "holding on" to their patients, sustaining the patient through times of danger. Beyond the positive emotional outcomes, physiological outcomes are also improved. Such salutogenic mutuality also changes the nurse. It is often a potent factor for developing the reservoir of resilience upon which critical care nurses must draw for long-term wellness and thriving.

This results from two functions of salutogenic experiences, a sense of coherence and meaning-making. When experiences in the critical care setting deepen a nurse's sense of life coherence and meaning, emotional resilience and capability deepen. Because of their deeply relational mechanism, grounded in interpersonal and communication capabilities, it is easy to recognize the contribution of EI abilities to these processes. For both emotional healing and development of salutogenic mutuality, EI abilities enhance performance, improve clinical outcomes, and support nurse thriving.

CRITICAL CARE RESEARCH AND EI

A body of critical care nursing EI research has just begun to develop. Early studies demonstrate correlations between EI and lower levels of ICU nurse perceived stress and burnout, and positive attitudes toward end of life care (Lewis, 2019; Munnangi et al., 2018; Park & Oh, 2019). Interventions to develop EI in critical care staff also correlate with staff wellness (Sharif et al., 2013).

DEVELOPING EMOTIONAL INTELLIGENCE IN CRITICAL CARE NURSING

EMOTIONAL INTELLIGENCE DEVELOPMENT SAMPLE EXERCISE #7: TELL ME A STORY

There is great power in telling the story. Salutogenic stories stay with us as nurses because they activate potent learning, or meaning, that informs us and makes us wise. Writing the stories down, or telling them to someone else, deepens the learning, and when needed, heals. Telling the story also develops abilities, reinforcing skills that were used, and developing those that were not. It solidifies learning and widens understanding. For these reasons, it can be useful to write down a story and identify what of the EI abilities were used, or not used, and how they might be used to greater effect in the future. The story is a teacher. The story is medicine.

REFERENCES

Lewis, S. L. (2019). Emotional intelligence in neonatal intensive care unit nurses: Decreasing moral distress in end-of-life care and laying a foundation for improved outcomes: An integrative review. *Journal of Hospice and Palliative Nursing, 21*(4), 250–256. https://doi.org/10.1097/NJH.0000000000000561

Mayer, J. D., Caruso, D., & Salovey, P. (1999). Emotional intelligence meets traditional standards for an intelligence. *Intelligence, 27,* 267–298. https://doi.org/10.1016/S0160-2896(99)00016-1

Munnangi, S., Dupiton, L., Boutin, A., & Angus, L. D. (2018). Burnout, perceived stress, and job satisfaction among trauma nurses at a level I safety net trauma center. *Journal of Trauma Nursing, 25,* 4–13. https://doi.org/10.1097/JTN.000000000000 0335

Park, J.-Y., & Oh, J. (2019). Influence of perceptions of death, end-of-life care stress, and emotional intelligence on attitudes towards end-of-life care. *Child Health Nursing Research, 25*(1), 38–47. https://doi.org/10.4094/chnr.2019.25.1.38

Sharif, F., Rezaie, S., Keshavarzi, S., Mansoori, P., & Ghadakpoor, S.(2013). Teaching emotional intelligence to intensive care unit nurses and their general health: A randomized clinical trial. *International Journal of Occupational and Environmental Medicine, 4*(3), 141–148.

8

Emotional Intelligence in Oncology Nursing

INTRODUCTION

Emotional intelligence (EI) is defined as the "ability to recognize the meanings of emotions .... and to reason and problem-solve on the basis of them" (Mayer et al., 1999, p. 267). In this chapter EI is operationalized with the following skills:

1. Accurate identification of emotions in self and others
*2. Understanding emotions
*3. Using emotions to reason (integrating thinking and feeling)
4. Managing emotions

For the purposes of this text, skills 2 and 3 are reversed from the order published in Mayer et al. (1999). This better aligns the EI abilities with the nursing process illustrated throughout this text. This chapter uses these skills as a framework to describe the use of EI abilities across the whole continuum of oncology care, from possibility of diagnosis to end-of-ife decision-making.

ONCOLOGY NURSING AND EI ABILITY

Across the continuum of care for patients with oncological disorders, emotional intelligence (EI) skills improve clinical outcomes, enhance nurse performance, and reduce risk. These abilities facilitate care that includes the following:

- oncology risk assessment,
- possible cancer diagnosis and new cancer diagnosis,

- active cancer treatment,
- symptom control,
- disease remission and disease recurrence,
- end-stage treatment and transition to terminal symptom control,
- withdrawal of treatment,
- hospice care, and
- engagement with grieving families.

The same EI abilities also support oncology nurses' care of themselves, their coworkers, and others on the care team. The physical, emotional, social, and spiritual labor required of oncology nursing makes EI abilities of particular importance. They improve patient safety, optimize patient outcomes, and develop resiliency (Codier et al., 2011).

EI and the Concept of Caring in Oncology Nursing

Oncology nursing differs from other specialty practice areas in several ways. First, each phase of care for oncology patients has its own unique emotional issues. Not only is each oncology patient's situation and experience unique, but that experience changes with each phase of treatment. Second, the nurse's relationship with their patients changes as their care evolves. Witnessing their patients' progress, successes, failures, disease endpoint, remission, and cure or death creates stresses, challenges, and opportunities for growth unique to oncology nursing. Third, cancer happens to families. Oncology nurses are constantly engaged with the patient's first line of support, who also have their own needs (Godfry, 2019).

Oncology nurses accompany patients on their cancer journey beginning with the possibility of a cancer diagnosis, through the long and tense process of diagnostic testing and biopsy staging. They help patients and their families choose treatments that have implications for self-image, relationships, finances, and future abilities. They witness emotional ups and downs, disease exacerbation and remission, cycles of hope and despair. In terminal care, nurses support last wishes as a patient's life journey ends. In these precious, life-affirming, difficult, and tender decisions, nurses are both healers and advocates.

Perhaps nowhere in nursing is caring so intrinsic to professional practice as it is in oncology nursing. But because caring is not behaviorally specific or measurable, this guiding star of oncology nursing remains ill-defined. EI abilities offer a way to conceptually operationalize and tangibly measure this important concept, making it easier to evaluate and improve (Codier, 2019).

Clinical Performance

In oncology care, clinical performance is particularly essential for patient safety and optimum clinical outcomes. Nursing performance influences cancer outcomes directly, through compliance with treatment regimen, sustainability of wellness habits that correlate with treatment survival, and cultivation of support systems to sustain the patient through treatment. Research findings demonstrate a correlation between EI ability with nurse clinical performance. So, developing oncology nurse EI ability may have a direct effect on oncology patients' clinical outcomes.

Interpersonal Relationships

Whether in the crucible of therapeutic relationships, teaching patients and their families, in collegial relationships that sustain and develop practice, or in interprofessional relationships, interpersonal relationship skill is crucial for oncology nurse practice. These capabilities also influence relationships within the oncology team and in nurses' own support systems. Research evidence, in nursing and other disciplines, correlates EI ability with interpersonal relationship efficacy. For this reason, development of EI abilities is an important way for oncology nurses to develop and maintain interpersonal effectiveness, improving both patient care and self-care.

Safety

Patient safety is most important when patients are most vulnerable, and oncology patients are particularly vulnerable across several risk categories. Older oncology patients may have preexisting fragile bones and skin, as well as age-related immune suppression. Cancer therapy adds to this baseline of risk. Compromised nutrition, therapy-induced immunosuppression, and multiple hospital and out-patient visits also add risk. Cancer therapy administration errors are uncommon, but given the potential toxicity of these agents, oncology medical errors are potentially devastating.

There is little research on EI ability and patient safety, but it is estimated that 80% of all medical errors are related to errors in communication (Kohn, 2000). Given the important role of communication and the established mediating role of EI in effective communication, improved EI ability could enhance effective communication and therefore the safety of oncology patients. This is one way to reduce clinical risk of all kinds, and to reduce vulnerability, in this high-risk population.

Burnout, Resilience, Emotional Labor, Career Longevity and Moral Distress

Oncology nurses are at particularly high risk for the negative effects of stress, burnout, emotional labor, and moral distress. Emotional resiliency, self-care, and preventive wellness skills are critical for these nurses. Although a great deal has been written on this subject, there is no good evidence for specific skills that prevent burnout, mitigate emotional labor, assist in processing moral distress, and facilitate relationships and practices that support oncology nurse thriving.

However, ample evidence shows the positive role of EI ability in mitigating negative emotional factors that can potentially compromise care and caregiver wellness (see references in Chapter 15). There is also preliminary evidence for use of EI development to enhance oncology nurses' emotional capabilities (Codier et al., 2013). No data is available on the impact of EI on burnout rates, retention on the job, and career longevity in the oncology nurse population. In the general nursing population, however, several subsets of EI ability correlate with retention in nurses' current job and total anticipated career length in a general nursing population (Codier et al., 2009), and extensive literature exists outside of nursing that supports the mitigating effect of EI on perceived stress and burnout, both in nursing and other disciplines.

Interprofessional Practice

Effective interprofessional practice is one of the keys to effective oncology care, yet evidence-based methods for measuring and improving interprofessional practice outcomes are lacking. Because EI ability correlates with general team effectiveness in other disciplines, such correlations certainly apply to interprofessional practice in oncology care as well. For oncology teams, where ethical and moral dilemmas are often processed within the context of the interdisciplinary team, the ability to identify, understand, use, and manage emotions may influence team success. Effective consensus and conflict resolution similarly may depend on team EI abilities.

APPLYING EI TO ONCOLOGY PRACTICE

EI abilities can improve performance and outcomes in many aspects of oncology nursing. How then do EI abilities specifically apply to oncology clinical practice?

Story: A Sad, *Sad* Day ... (From the Journal of an EI Nurse Researcher)

Using EI: Identifying Emotions

The unit was one of the clinical sites for a research project on EI in clinical oncology. An inpatient oncology unit at a large urban tertiary care center, oncology patients across the whole continuum of oncology care received testing for possible cancer diagnoses, initial cancer treatment, management of acute complications or acute symptoms, and terminal end-of-life care. The nursing staff was sharp, committed, involved, and interested in learning, but the psychological care of the patients was problematic. They did not identify emotional problems in this population at high risk for emotional disturbances, and a chart review of six months of care revealed not a single case of emotional problem-solving. EI was selected as a framework for beginning to address this problem.

The research study was simple. Once a week, the research team of three nurses, an oncology APRN, a staff nurse, and a nurse researcher did "EI Rounds." Over the course of the rounds, the team spoke with a few nurses on the unit, one at a time. The team asked two questions: "What is your patient feeling today?" and after that, "What are you feeling today?" These questions had been selected because the study was based on the four-branch ability model in which identification of emotions was the first step. As an exploratory study, the research team thought these questions would be a good place to begin.

After several weeks, the researchers noticed the staff was competing to participate in the EI rounds. Clinical research is limited if staff are too busy or do not value clinical research, but in this case, the staff were fighting over the chance to participate. "No, it is my turn ... you did last week!" This was not a variable measured in the study, but anecdotally it appeared that the nurses were very eager to be asked how they felt.

Despite this, the research team quickly recognized the nurses, who were all intelligent, well-educated, caring, and professional nurses, had difficulty answering the questions, "What is your patient feeling, and what are you feeling?" Responses like, "Fine," or, "The patient is going home," and, "Busy," were common, none of which are emotions! Even though the nurses seemed very eager to be asked about their emotions, a large percentage of responses had nothing to do with emotions at all. These were not unintelligent nurses. When reminded that "fine" and "busy" are not emotions, they laughed and agreed. The staff, it appeared, was not in the habit of identifying emotions in themselves or their patients. This on an oncology unit, where acute states of fear, anxiety, dread, hopelessness, and pain were encountered daily.

Then came the phone call. The research team had identified an ethical problem with the research study and told me they needed to see me right away. We sat down together, and I asked, "What happened?" The team members said when they arrived on the unit that day, they encountered a group of nurses in the nurses' station. The research team greeted them casually, and the group responded, "It is a sad day. It is a sad, *sad* day." Without prompting or artifice, several of the nurses shook their heads and agreed, "a sad day." A well-loved patient had unexpectedly died, and a new patient with a particularly bad prognosis was recently admitted. Unprompted, uncoordinated, completely unselfconsciously, "sad" kept coming up, over and over again. "It is a sad, *sad* day."

The research team emphasized to me they had never heard the staff talk like this. This was a huge breakthrough they attributed to the EI rounds. What sounded simple actually reflected a profound shift. I asked expectantly, "And the ethical problem?" Their response stunned me. They believed the EI rounds had affected the unit so profoundly, it was unethical to withhold it from the other shifts and other units. They suggested the research study be stopped and the EI rounds be immediately implemented in all units in the hospital. All because we asked, "What is your patient feeling today? What are you feeling?"

Story Reflection

The team finished the study. As an exploratory study, it left the team with as many questions as answers. Some findings were not surprising. Nurses who could not identify their own emotions also could not name their patients' emotions. As the study progressed, identification and documentation for emotional patient problem-solving improved significantly. Other findings were more surprising, such as the degree of maladaptive emotional processing reported by the nurses, such as, "I just try not to think about it," or "After a rough day I just go home and eat too much." The nurses' evaluations of EI rounds varied in degree but not in type. Of the nurses who participated in the study, 100% reported the rounds were helpful to some degree. The power of simply naming emotions stunned the research team. "What are you feeling today?" (Codier et al., 2013).

Applying EI

Using EI: Identifying and Understanding Emotions

Emotions, like elements listed on a traditional periodic table, have properties and characteristics. Like the elements found in nature, emotions can be active or passive. Some combine with others in predictable ways, changing, and transforming. Oncology nurses must be "emotion scientists" astutely identifying and understanding emotions in their patients, families, and in themselves.

For example, understanding grief is central to oncology practice. The importance of understanding grief throughout the continuum of oncology care is difficult to overstate. From the initial reality of losing a disease-free life, through phases of disease exacerbation and remission, to loss of physical capability and ultimate loss of life, oncology patients constantly grieve. It is intrinsic to cancer oncology nurses that they become masters of this territory, beginning with a deep and nuanced understanding of grief and the complex constellation of emotions that accompany it.

Most nurses learn in nursing school about the stages of grief. As oncology nurses gain experience, the depth and nuance of this understanding increases. Shock, anger, denial, bargaining, acceptance, and withdrawal are all part of the grieving process, but these stages are not linear. Patients cycle back and forth between these emotions and their emotional processes evolve as they do so. The patient who is angry one day may exhibit the dull emotional thickness of shock the next, and as quickly experience a new sense of acceptance the day after that. The grieving process is cyclic, organic, influenced by many factors, and is highly personal.

The implications of understanding the varied colors, shades, and nuances of grief in oncology practice are endless. The experience of grief varies among oncology patients. For one patient, the loss of time with grandchildren may be more powerful than loss of years of their own life. For another, the end of learning may be the focus of grief. For patients receiving chemotherapy, hair loss could be an issue of visual aesthetics, self-image, vanity, sexuality, or just hating hats! The ability to apply an understanding of grief and its related emotions, the transformation of one emotion into another, and the aggregate effects of emotions (like emotional pain, frustration, exhaustion, and despair) require EI abilities.

Understanding the impact of grief on patient learning is also important. When teaching a patient whose early stages of grieving has strong elements of shock, simple information, repeated regularly, may be needed. But for a patient experiencing the anger stage, simplicity and repetition could be infuriating. For a patient beginning to emotionally detach, very common in advanced stages of grieving, information others deem important may not seem so to the patient. For these reasons, identifying emotions in the various stages of grief and understanding the impact of grief on learning is crucial for patient teaching that is offered to grieving patients and their families. Using EI abilities to assess and emotionally problem-solve may be necessary before any learning can be effective.

Using EI: Using Emotions to Reason

When emotions are used in a "think/feel" process, integrating emotion and reasoning, reasoning informs feelings and feelings informs reasoning. Using this EI ability, engagement with a patient's emotional experience or one's own, gains nuance and depth. When teaching a grieving patient, a nurse weaves identification and understanding of the patient's emotions with what the nurse understands about grief. Out of this think/feel process, a deeper and more comprehensive plan for teaching can be developed. Using emotions to reason can also help prevent emotional errors, which can occur when an emotion is misidentified or understood incorrectly as it applies to a given situation.

Story: Trying to Die

A novice inpatient hospice nurse, upset and in distress, made an appointment to meet with the unit nurse manager immediately. Once in the nurse manager's office, the young nurse pulled her hand out of her pocket and emptied a small handful of pills, narcotics, onto the table between them. She said, "I found them in my patient's drawer, hidden in a sock. I took the sock out of the drawer, thinking it needed laundering and accidentally found them."

The nurse manager, an advanced practice nurse and long-time nurse expert in end-of-life care, watched the young nurse. "Why did you take them?" she asked before calmly adding, "What is your concern?"

The young nurse flushed and looked up angrily. "He could kill himself, that is why. He is obviously stockpiling narcotics. I was worried. Aren't you?"

The nurse manager smiled gently. She affirmed the young nurse for her care of the patient and said, "You are right, I am worried, but for a different reason. Can you think of any other reason why he might be saving medications?" After the young nurse looked at her blankly, the manager continued, "Patients do sometimes stockpile medications to end their life. Usually just knowing they have that option gives them a sense of control. Sometimes just that control gives them peace. You and I should talk more about that another time because it is clear you have strong feelings about that. But what I am worried about right now is this man's pain control. How are we doing with that?"

The nurse reported pain control had been difficult, but recently, the patient's pain was finally under good control. "He had a hard time for the first couple of days. His pain was pretty bad." The nurse manager waited, her face expectant, as the young nurse thought for a few minutes. Finally, she said, "Oh, no. What if he was saving medications in case his pain got bad again? What if he doesn't trust us to control his pain? What if that is why he saved his meds, so he could control his pain if we don't?"

The nurse manager smiled and nodded. "I agree with you. My biggest concern is that he undermedicated himself so he could save the pills in case he needed them later. Maybe he did save medications because he does not trust us. *That* is what I am worried about." The two nurses, elder and younger, put their heads together and talked for a long time, making a plan to address restoration of trust between their patient and the team trying to care for him.

Story: Take a Nap! (From an Interview With a Nurse Educator, Used With Permission)

I think it is really important people don't assume they identify emotions correctly. I am really close to my students and they often come to me for advice. Just about once a semester, a student comes to my office distraught and in tears. 'Professor, I am depressed. Should I see a psychiatrist and get on medication?'

I always say the same thing, 'Maybe you do need that, and I will help you find the help you need if that is the case. But let me ask you, when is the last time you slept?'

At this point, the student invariably looks at me blankly, and answers with some variation of, 'Well, I have had to go in really early to prepare for clinical, and you know we had that really hard test this week, and, well, I have barely slept.'

Students do not understand that depression and acute fatigue feel very similar emotionally. Particularly at the end of the semester when the cumulative fatigue hits them, students get mentally fatigued enough that they can't perceive the difference. So we sit down and have a talk about that, and plan. I emphasize that student services could help them connect with a psychiatrist and anti-depressive medication if needed. But when I follow up with these students, invariably they report they realized they didn't need a pill ... they needed a nap! Exhaustion and depression look and feel a lot alike, but the difference between them is huge! Their causes and treatment differ so accurate identification is critical. Oncology patients, for whom fatigue and depression are frequent, must be able to accurately identify the difference between these two emotions.

Reflection on These Stories

Both these stories illustrate that managing emotions depends on identifying, understanding, and using emotions to reason. In the first story, the despair that the novice nurse assumed was driving her patient's behavior was, in fact, mistrust. If the patient's mistrust had not been identified correctly, the team's intervention (taking over control and setting limits to "protect" the patient) could have made the patient's mistrust worse, creating a vicious cycle. Once the novice nurse's mentor helped her identify the emotional state of her patient accurately, she could make a plan that could address the real emotion underlying the patient's behavior. In the second story, misidentification of simple fatigue could have resulted in unnecessary medication.

How to Manage Emotions

One way to think about managing emotions is what Dr. Marc Brackett calls "emotional regulation" (Brackett, 2019). This is not about controlling, repressing, or denying emotions or setting aside an emotion like an obstructive piece of furniture. To manage or regulate an emotion is to work with it, not against it, to problem-solve. This is what characterizes an emotion scientist, one who is responding intentionally to emotions they identify, understand, use, and manage. This is vastly different from emotional reactivity, which is a rapid reaction without thought or consideration. Managing emotions may simply mean choosing a new course of action. It could be saying to a friend, "I am too upset about what you said to respond now. Our relationship is important to me, so let me think about this and get back to you later." It could be a plan for self-care, "I am exhausted! I need to rest before I think this problem through," or plan for an energizing activity amid an emotional challenge. What makes this EI skill effective is its foundation in identifying emotions accurately, understanding them, and using them to reason.

RESEARCH FINDINGS: EI AND SELF-CARE FOR ONCOLOGY NURSES

The correlation between EI and nurse stress, burnout, and coping are particularly relevant for oncology nurses (Ebstein et al., 2019). One study demonstrated a significant relationship between oncology nurses' measured EI and problem-focused coping, and an inverse relationship between EI and occupational stress (Espinoza & Sanhueza, 2012). In another, there was a negative correlation between fear of death and EI in nursing students working with oncology patients (Espinoza & Sanhueza, 2012). In a group of inpatient oncology nurses, ability to identify their own emotions correlated with ability to identify their patient's emotions (Codier et al.,

2013). In a study of breast cancer survivors, measured EI predicted health-related quality of life (Mirzaei et al., 2019).

DEVELOPING EMOTIONAL INTELLIGENCE ABILITIES

SAMPLE EMOTIONAL INTELLIGENCE DEVELOPMENT EXERCISE #8: THE FORMULA

Difficult interpersonal confrontations are problematic because of the ease with which such encounters can degenerate into judging, blaming, and persistent negative emotions. One suggestion is to use "The formula." To use it, fill in the blanks. When you _____, I feel _____. What I would like to ask is _____. For example: "When you roll your eyes when I talk, I feel put down. What I would like to ask is that you don't do that when we are talking." Or, "When you rush me through report, I have trouble organizing my thoughts. What I want to ask is that you be patient with me so I can give a good report."

REFERENCES

Brackett, M. (2019). *Permission to feel. Celadon books.* Macmillan Publishers.

Codier, E. (2019). Emotional intelligence in oncology nursing. In J. K. Payne & K. Murphe-Ende (Eds.), *Current trends in oncology nursing* (2nd ed.). Oncology Nursing Society.

Codier, E., Kamikawa, C., Kooker, B. M., & Shoultz, J. (2009). Emotional intelligence, performance, and retention in clinical staff nurses. *Nursing Administration Quarterly, 33*(4), 310–316. https://doi.org/10.1097/NAQ.0b013e3181b9dd5d

Codier, E., Muneno, L., & Freitas, E. (2011). Emotional intelligence abilities in oncology and palliative care. *Journal of Hospice and Palliative Care Nursing, 13*(3), 183–188. https://doi.org/10.1097/NJH.0b013e31820ce14b

Codier, E., Muneno, L., & Freitas, E. (2013). Emotional intelligence rounds: Developing emotional intelligence ability in clinical oncology nurses. *Oncology Nurse Forum, 40*(1), 22–29. https://doi.org/10.1188/13.ONF.22-29

Ebstein, A. M., Sanzero, L., See Tan, K., Cherniss, C., Ruggeiro, J., & Cimiotti, J. (2019). The relationships between coping, occupational stress, and emotional intelligence in newly hired oncology nurses. *Psycho-Oncology, 28*(2), 278–283. https://doi.org/10.1002/pon.4937

Espinoza, V., & Olivia Sanhueza, A. (2012). Fear of death and its relationship with emotional intelligence of nursing students in Concepción. *ACTA Paulista de Enfermagem, 25*(4), 607–613.

Godfry, N. (2019). Professional identity, image and insights in career planning. In J. K. Payne & K. Murphe-Ende (Eds.), *Current trends in oncology nursing* (2nd ed., pp. 423–434). Oncology Nurses Society.

Kohn, L. T., Corrigan, J. M., & Donaldson, M. S. (Eds.). (2000). *To err is human: Building a safer health system*. Quality Chasm Series. National Academies Press. https://www.nap.edu/catalog/9728/toerrishumanbuildingasaferhealth system

Mayer, J. D., Caruso, D., & Salovey, P. (1999). Emotional intelligence meets traditional standards for an intelligence. *Intelligence, 27*, 267–298. https://doi.org/10.1016/S0160-2896(99)00016-1

Mirzaei, S., Tame, A. I., & Anbiaie, R. (2019). Emotional intelligence as a predictor of health-related quality of life in breast cancer survivors. *Asia-Pacific Journal of Oncology Nursing, 6*(3), 261–268. https://doi.org/10.4103/apjon.apjon_76_18

9

Emotional Intelligence and Nursing Education

INTRODUCTION

In this chapter, the four EI abilities, identifying emotions, understanding them, using them to reason, and managing, are applied to nursing education (Mayer et al., 1999). Their usual order is adapted to best align with the nursing process. Situated cognition theory is presented as a theoretical foundation for the integration of EI into nursing education practice.

NURSING SCHOOL AND EMOTIONAL INTELLIGENCE

Story: Deaf, Mute, and Blind

When the nurse remembered her first pediatric patient in nursing school, she recalled a child less than one year of age admitted to the hospital for a systemic infection. The nurse could see clearly in her mind the sight of the child laying flaccid in bed, moving occasionally to touch, staring in no particular direction, eyes open but unseeing. This child had been born deaf, blind, and mute. She remembered the parents, hovering. They leaned over the bed, rarely sitting, as if ready to take action, if only they could find some action to take. This was the first pediatric rotation assignment for this nurse, her first experience of caring for an ill child.

That day, the nurse went back to her dorm room after clinical. She listened to the rock opera, "Tommy," a song about another deaf, mute, and blind child. She played the song over and over, trying to wrap her mind and heart around what life could be for her patient. What could she, as a nurse, possibly do for the child's agonized parents? What is nursing care, and being a nurse, in the face of tragedy like that?

The nurse does not remember anything about her pediatric nursing instructor, not on that difficult day nor on any other day of the semester.

Man or woman? Tall or short? Mean or nice? No images or impressions came to mind. The clinical instructor was completely absent from this nurse's memory of one of the most potent, life-changing, seminal days of her nursing career. Probably the instructor was there, doing something. Maybe the instructor shrugged and said, "That student is doing fine."

Applying EI to the Emotional Education of Student Nurses

When students process affective events in clinical experiences, they are not just applying course material. Clinical experiences as just described present students with highly emotionally charged, personal experiences. Students learn to experience and process their emotions witnessing suffering, death, and family struggles. These emotional learning experiences are among the most important in nursing education and act as crucibles within which students form professionally. They offer students a chance to grow in wisdom, resilience, and emotional capability. Clinical instructors offer mentoring, role modeling, and support during these seminal experiences. Without their guidance, students may be traumatized or form negative emotional patterns. They may fall into habits of emotional disengagement and emotional constriction or deprioritizing of emotional care. These constitute risk factors for poor performance, compassion fatigue, interpersonal distancing, and burnout.

However, early experiences like those in the story can also lead to transformative, seminal learning. Across their professional lives, nurses inevitably come into close contact with grief, death, sadness, tragedy, suffering, and a host of other emotional challenges. These emotions are not just a problem to overcome or endure. Rather, they offer an opportunity for deep learning. Witnessing grief, for example, offers students a chance to develop a broader understanding as they learn to embrace the unexpected gifts that grief experiences can offer. If students do not learn to identify the emotions they encounter in challenging clinical situations, they miss an opportunity for transformative learning.

But what of instructor skills? The absence of the instructor in the student's story suggests that they maintained an emotional distance from the student. It is possible the instructor lacked the emotional skills necessary to do anything else. This is not uncommon. Most preparation for clinical educators does not include development of abilities to guide students in the development of their own emotional skills. The master's essentials curriculum document which guides their education barely mentions them. The emotional intelligence (EI) abilities could provide a structure for such skill development, providing clinical instructors a means to improve their own student interactions. This could make clinical instructors more effective teachers, mentors, and coaches.

Using EI: Identifying Emotions

Failure to identify difficult emotions places a nurse at professional risk. No nurse plans to burn out, becoming emotionally detached or distant, unable to offer compassionate care. So, how does this happen? One seminal cause is failure to identify challenging emotions correctly. When a nurse identifies a traumatic emotional response accurately, they can intentionally activate their self-care reserves or ask for help. This runs counter to the prevailing medical culture of emotional denial and detachment. The false assumption that strong feelings cloud objectivity and contaminate reasoning costs patients and caregivers alike. Nurses must learn to do the hard work of emotional integration, beginning with identifying their own emotions accurately.

For the student caring for the deaf, blind, and mute child, what emotions would it have been important for the nursing student to identify in themselves, their patient, and the child's parents?

Students must be taught to check their identification of emotions to ensure they are accurate. It is hazardous to assume people identify emotions correctly. Consider the scenario of a seriously injured child admitted to the hospital ER. The parents appear to be overcome with grief and worry for their child and the nurse assumes this is true. But what if the parents are abusive and caused the child's injury? What appears to be grief and worry, may instead be guilt and apprehension. In this case, misidentification of an emotion could place the child at risk.

When Emotions Are Not Identified: The Cost of Denial

As well as limiting emotional learning, denying or minimizing powerful emotions in emotionally charged situations undermines effective student performance. For example, if a student is struggling with sadness, it could interfere with care of the patient and family. Sadness takes up attention and energy needed to perform well. It can distract and delay responses in crisis and result in superficial or inaccurate assessment findings. Denying this emotion does not improve attention and performance, but rather prolongs its disruptive effects. Naming and briefly exploring the sadness may enable a student to move on, maintaining patient safety without distraction. This is true of any strong emotion that students encounter during clinical experiences. If they are taught to separate these emotions off from their care, patterns of emotional splintering, denial, and distancing can result.

Using EI: Understanding Emotions and Using Emotions to Reason

Understanding emotions, their nuance, physiological basis, and particular phenomenology is crucial for managing them effectively. The parents from the story illustrate the importance of understanding anxiety.

Anxiety is an emotion that involves the release of adrenalin. Physiologically, this results in a hypermetabolic state, elevated blood pressure, heart rate, and muscle tension. Activation of the fight/flight response makes an individual prone to restless movement and hyper-alerted states. Relaxing, even staying still, may prove difficult. The child's parents were unable to sit and simply be with their child as a result of their anxiety. This behavior is physically exhausting. By identifying and understanding this anxiety response, the nursing student could have used this information to reason, thinking about how to help the parents manage anxiety in a way that does not exhaust them.

Using EI: Managing Emotions

Accurately identifying and understanding emotions, and using them to reason, offers nurses specific ways to manage emotionally difficult situations. This applies to care of patients but also to self-care. In the story, changing the parents' hovering behavior might have helped them conserve energy and improve interpersonal interactions with each other and their child. It could also provide an opportunity to address other ways for them to conserve their energy. The student might identify their own sadness and grief for their patient and, understanding its potential for undermining performance, might plan to call on a friend or set aside reflection time later in the day. Reflecting on the experience and sharing it with others could mitigate its negative effects and deepen learning.

APPLYING EI ABILITIES IN HOSPITAL NURSING EDUCATION

As well as using EI in nursing school, EI abilities can also be used by clinical mentors, unit CNS, and nurse educators to support the unique emotional learning needs of unit orientees and staff.

Story: Burn Death

The novice nurse was orienting to the Burn Unit and was paired with one of the unit's most experienced nurses. Their assignment for the day was a young man with black charred burns across most of his body. His eyes were swollen shut and facial burns rendered him nearly unrecognizable. His hands were the only part of his body that could be touched safely. He lay alone on the bed. No family or friends were present. As his death was inevitable, his treatment consisted of only comfort care. The orientee's preceptor carefully talked through the care goals and anticipated events. She calmly described the electrolyte imbalance that would soon end his life. What the orientee noticed most was her gentleness and patience, with both the orientee's learning and their patient's terrible, inevitable death.

Soon the two nurses noticed the EKG changes presaging their patient's death. The mentor sat down beside their patient and quietly spoke to him, "Your body is too burned to live, and you will die very soon. Don't be afraid. I am on this side, and I won't leave you. And God is on the other side, and won't leave you, either." She held his hand until his EKG flatlined. Wordlessly, she gave her orientee a hug, turned to a window next to their patient's bed, and opened it as if to let his spirit fly into the clear dark night. Mentor and orientee stood at the window together before closing it and returning to his bedside to prepare his body for the morgue.

Applying EI

Mentoring, because of its intrinsic interpersonal context, is rich with possibility for applying EI abilities to improve orientee learning, performance, and longevity. The mentor in this story used EI to give better care, support deep learning, and at the same time develop nurse resilience and longevity.

Using EI: Identifying Emotions

The mentor was clearly aware of the emotions in herself, her orientee, and, to the extent possible, her patient. Her patient was at the end of life. His injuries made it impossible for him to express himself or even acknowledge he could hear. An assessment of his emotions was impossible, but given the patient's experience of the fire, emergency intervention, transport to the burn unit, and the voices of those around him, it was likely that if conscious, he was at least anxious. Fear of death was likely.

The mentor was also aware of the feelings of the novice nurse she was orienting. Just seeing the burns is traumatic for novice burn nurses and the horror and revulsion that is common can impair both learning and job performance. When critical care priorities shift from aggressive life-saving measures to comfort and terminal care, the process can be both challenging and traumatic for staff. What was the mentor feeling? A dying man and a totally green novice to deal with at the same time! One can only imagine the emotions that the mentor was aware of in herself.

Using EI: Understanding Emotions and Using Emotions to Reason

As a mature mentor, she knew traumatic emotions undermine performance and learning, putting a novice at long-term performance and burnout risk. She also knew that if her patient was conscious, it would only be for a short time. She had only minutes to help him face the last moments of his life. By understanding the complex emotions this acute clinical situation presented, the mentor was able to use emotions to reason, both of which were needed to emotionally problem-solve in this difficult situation.

Using EI: Managing Emotions

This nurse's EI maturity enabled her to choose appropriate actions for her patient and at the same time support an orientee facing a new and challenging experience. She offered the dying man information, comfort, and presence as he died. At the same time, she supported the orientee's learning by managing the complex system of emotions flowing through this experience. What about opening the window, something rarely done in a burn ICU? Those few moments with the orientee, looking out into the night together, taking a minute, taking a breath, offering a hug for reassurance, demonstrated emotional embracing and life-affirmation that modeled self-care for effective learning and long-term thriving.

APPLYING EI TO REIMAGINE NURSING EDUCATION

Invitation to a Revolution

In 1961, nursing theorist Martha Rogers wrote a seminal text called *Education Revolution in Nursing*, in which she called for a radically new approach to nursing education (Rogers, 1961). This call still resonates 60 years later as many of the challenges she identified remain, yet little change has occurred. In most nursing schools, students still sit passively in rows, in long class periods (not uncommonly three or four hours), and watch PowerPoint slides, one after another, as the teacher, in "sage-on-stage" mode, dispenses information. A "wink, wink, nod, nod" contract exists between teacher and student. The teacher is expected to create and distribute a PowerPoint presentation of material that will be covered on the test. Students, who largely multitask during these classes, regurgitate required information on exams that by default define their mastery of the material. The format of such tests is almost invariably multiple choice or what students refer as "multiple guess." This emphasizes content recall over critical thinking or problem-solving. No one thinks that students would be able to achieve the same grade if the test was readministered even a week later, and test achievement has no correlation with content application in a clinical setting, graduation rates, or professional achievement after school. "Wink, wink, nod, nod. Let's all agree this is education."

Grade point average and class standing do not correlate with graduation rate, NCLEX pass rate, or performance post-graduation. Little data support standardized testing for prediction of nursing school performance and many nursing schools no longer use them for admission screening criteria. Nursing student burnout and burnout rates in the first year of employment after graduation are high. Students often leave within the first two years, creating a combined tragedy of dashed personal and professional hopes and financial investment loss for the schools and hospitals. The top-performing nursing graduates do not go on to be the top-performing, resilient, and enduring nurses.

Simulation as a bridge technology between didactic learning and clinical practice has improved student outcomes. This approach has been successful for several reasons that hold a key to the future of nursing education and reveal an important role for EI abilities. Simulation learning is predicated philosophically on the theory of distributed cognition, which focuses on learning as a socially contextualized process interconnected with context, culture, and relationships. Simulation learning also incorporates emotions, emotional phenomena, and emotional interpersonal dynamics in the learning process. This offers an opportunity, even unintentionally, to integrate EI abilities in the learning process and to develop EI abilities across the simulation experience. Foundational to these changes is a dramatic shift in how nurses are taught clinical reasoning. In words that summarize research findings about the role of EI in clinical reasoning, one researcher concluded, "Continuing to separate cognition and emotion in research, theorizing and scholarship on clinical reasoning is counterproductive" (Hutchinson et al., 2017, p. 4).

Envisioning the Problem: The Brain in a Bottle

Picture an empty classroom with rows of typical college classroom chairs. A crystal glass jar full of a clear fluid sits on the writing desk arm of each chair. Inside each jar is a brain, alive, pulsating, taking in what it is "fed" from the speaker at the front of the room. This classroom full of brains sitting in their jars, each self-contained, taking in and processing information independently, closed off from others. Nursing students continue to be taught as if this is how learning occurs.

This individualistic, dualistic, disembodied model of learning teaches students to operate as solo practitioners. Although nursing school performance criteria reference nursing teams and interprofessional practice, they reflect little actual skill-building or team competence. Collaboration, consensus building, conflict management, and resolution of ethical dilemmas might be touched upon. However, for the most part, these skills are neither taught nor evaluated, and no baseline competency is required.

To change this, nurse educators must think differently and students must learn to learn differently. The first step is to change ideas about cognition.

Thinking Differently About Thinking: The Theory of Distributed Cognition

Nursing education has begun to evolve toward a very different model of cognition based on the theory of distributed cognition. This theory suggests that all effective and deep learning results from a complex interweaving of being, doing, and interacting within a wide range of contexts. In this system, the learner is part of a vast social, cultural, emotional, and physical network that includes other people, social and cultural contexts, and electronic networks. Texting, Instagram, social media platforms, and other web-based communication systems are recognized as part of the cognition system. In contrast to the isolated "brain in a jar," learning, this system is dynamic. It evolves and transforms both the learner and the entire system simultaneously (Sutton, 2006). Nursing students not only learn in dyads and groups, but in a rich, interconnected physical, cultural, and electronic system that becomes not only their classroom but effectively their own extended neural network. Freed from its glass jar, cognition is distributed across this network. Sharing critical thinking and emotional problem-solving this way, collaboration is not just permitted, it is required.

If explicitly adopted, this model has staggering implications for nursing education and provides a theoretical context for use of EI in nursing education. This approach is dramatically different, both functionally and philosophically, from traditional nursing education. Given that all knowledge is situated in a physical, social, and cultural context, nursing education must be context focused. Additionally, it must shift away from fact-based empiricism and mind-body dualism. This approach also presents a very different power structure. Traditional education is a pyramid of power with the instructor at the top and students at the bottom. Distributed cognition places students firmly at the center of learning. Both power and responsibility for learning are not for the teacher to dispense, but for students to own.

Sample: Distributed Cognition in Nursing Education—Clinical Rounds in Virtual Space

In one exploratory study, students were taught graduate-level pathophysiology, and learning outcomes were measured in a three-dimensional virtual world. Instead of the usual, "read-the-book, take-the-test," approach, students, in electronic avatar form on their own computers at home, did hospital clinical rounds with a small group of their peers (also present in their avatar form). Course content mastery was measured by students' participation in rounds and graded by analysis of an electronic transcript of the activity.

Each round's learning activity focused on a specific pathology that required study of both basic physiology and pathophysiology prior to the activity. The group of five or six students completing the roundsmet at the virtual hospital. The instructor was present for only the first rounds, as an orientation exercise. The students began rounds with a review of pertinent physiology and pathological changes of their patient's illness. Then, as a group, they interviewed their patient for that day to discover how the pathology had manifest in their patient's life. After the interview, the group, as a team, discussed the patient's condition and plan for care. This was not, "read the book, take the test." Students had to read the book, then demonstrate mastery of what they had learned in a clinical situation. Rounds also required team learning. Students shared knowledge and practiced working together to care for patients and their families. This made for multilayered learning. Each week, students were assigned a different role for rounds, including leader, evaluator, scheduler, and acting as the patient. Learning about content material, interview skills, collegial interaction, role performance, and emotional problem-solving happened all at once, creating multidimensional and deep learning experiences.

Students used a computer-generated, verbatim transcript of each 30-minute clinical rounds session to review and complete self, peer, and group evaluations. The instructor reviewed these evaluations and the exercise transcript to formulate feedback and learning activity grades for each student. Based on all this feedback, students set behavioral goals for the next learning activity, creating a continuous improvement cycle. Unlike most group activities, every student had to perform their role. With the learning activity transcript as evidence, no one could be carried by the group. Emotional data, emotional problem-solving, and emotional issues were included in both the performance and feedback systems. All this resulted in a level of evaluation and feedback not possible in traditional learning.

The research study summarized both individual and group learning outcomes. Outcomes were achieved at the 100% level over 90% of the time. Student participation, evaluated by the volume and content of each student's input on the transcripts, was shared more evenly than typical of most small-group learning activities. Student evaluations reported that shy students, students culturally uncomfortable with leader roles, or students for whom English was a second language, were all more active than they had been previously.

Varied and multilayered learning characterized this rich format. Course content was reviewed, applied, and shared. Ideas bounced back and forth about how it would be used in real-world situations. Professional roles became clearer as students interacted with other disciplines. Students also reported feeling completely immersed in the learning activity with no distractions or multitasking. One student called this "engrossment." Students described the learning as deep. They had a name for how the group worked through these scenarios together: the group brain. They began to include evaluation of the group brain in their learning activity review. "How did the group brain do this week?" they asked (Codier, 2016; Codier & Holt, 2012; Codier et al., 2014).

APPLYING EI TO LEARNING: DISTRIBUTED COGNITION

The kind of learning in the rounds exercise epitomizes distributed cognition. Students began rounds by reviewing course content relevant to rounds that day, "What do we know about risks for heart disease in general and in women specifically?" They then approached these facts in context by discussing what they knew about their patient's life, circumstances, emotional issues, and culture/belief systems alongside the presentation and progression of their disease. After interacting with the patient, they had additional information that enabled them as a group to use the "group brain" to process as a team, and together formulate a plan of care. This learning activity also demonstrates the role of emotions, emotional content, emotional problem-solving, and emotional interactions as integral to learning.

Using EI: Identifying Emotions

During rounds, students improved learning and performance by being able to identify emotions that affected their learning. During the transcript review of one patient assessment, one student noticed a poor flow of communication. They realized the patient had brought up an uncomfortable subject, and the student, in order to emotionally avoid it, changed the subject at a critical juncture. The student's ability to identify how their feelings shut down the flow of important information was crucial in improving their performance in future interviews. This "ah-ha!" learning was immediate, powerful, and deep.

Similarly, reviewing transcripts often helped students to identify patient emotions accurately. During one rounds interview, the patient reported escalating chest pain. While reviewing the transcript of a rounds interview, students realized their interview style had created stress for the patient. In this case, failure to identify the patient's emotional state resulted in a deterioration of their clinical condition. Such a personal experience of realizing that the team's intervention had a negative impact was potent learning for the group that they were not likely to ever forget!

Using EI: Understanding Emotions

Learning based on distributed cognition, as in the rounds activity, helps students understand emotions better. In one virtual group discussion, the exercise goal was to use the three phases of consensus formation (brainstorming, finding themes, formulating consensus) to achieve group consensus on a clinical ethical problem. After students reviewed the activity transcript, many identified that in particular phases of consensus, they consistently monopolized the discussion. Their excitement and over-participation prevented others from contributing. This understanding of the relationship between excitement, hyper-verbal behavior, and excluding others was key to improving their performance. In evaluations, comments like, "I will not be such an air hog next time. I will ask others what they are thinking," were common. In other ethical discussions, students could identify their own negative emotional reactions when confronted with challenging ideas. Understanding the interpersonal dynamics that this created helped students change behavior and build better collegial and team relationships.

Using EI: Using Emotions to Reason

In learning activities based on distributed cognition, students have a great opportunity to use their emotions to reason. In one virtual clinical rounds activity, the group observed subtle hostile verbal behavior in their patient. In the group reflection, they all reported feeling nervous and fearful, unsure of how to interpret and respond to the behavior. The group then reviewed the activity transcript. Using both the written data and their reflections on their feelings at the time, they used their feelings to inform what they were thinking, and their thinking about the situation informed the feelings they had experienced. This changed their assessment of the patient and the resulting care plan. This also changed students' self-assessments, as they realized their feelings in response to the patient were not only normal, but that identifying their emotions was crucial for accurate patient assessment. The students realized their emotions represented important information.

Using EI: Managing Emotions

Through review and analysis of an interview of a hostile patient having chest pain, the students learned to manage emotions better. They helped the patient understand that his anger and hostility was worsening his chest pain. They validated his anger but also helped him focus on relaxing and resolving his chest pain. As a group, the students were able to focus on managing their own emotional responses to the patient's hostility. While reviewing the transcript, one student identified that they all felt defensive, and in response, they had effectively "ganged up on" the patient, which caused both his anger and his chest pain to worsen! The learning activity offered students a powerful opportunity to learn new approaches to managing anger in themselves, in patients, and as a group.

NURSING EDUCATION AND EI RESEARCH

Research on Nursing Students

Findings from EI education research across all disciplines is convincing. A 2019 meta-analysis of over 42,000 students from almost 160 research studies across numerous disciplines concluded that EI correlated with academic success (MacCann et al., 2019). A substantial body of nursing research validates this finding in the nursing student population (see summary in Chapter 15). In summary, in addition to evidence for positive correlation between EI and academic success, there is evidence of correlation of student EI with clinical performance, critical thinking, peer learning, appropriate assistance requests, professionalism, psychological resilience, interpersonal abilities, physical and emotional well-being, interpersonal skill level, problem-focused coping, problem-solving, and perceived competency. Negative correlations are demonstrated with perceived nursing student stress. Measured nursing student EI correlates with nursing program completion and NCLEX pass rate (Rode & Brown, 2019). In a 2014 study of success in nursing school, the EI of over 300 nursing students was predictive of arguably the three most important measures of nursing school success: academic performance, clinical performance, and program completion (Rankin, 2013).

In the general EI literature, broad evidence demonstrates that EI can be improved with a wide variety of interventions. This is summarized in a 2018 systematic review of 46 research studies investigating this subject (Kotsou et al., 2018). Evidence in the nursing research literature has demonstrated that student EI can be improved using methods as varied as standardized EI education, reflective writing, video training, and group reflective discussion (see summary of this research in Chapter 15).

DEVELOPING EMOTIONAL INTELLIGENCE ABILITIES

DEVELOPING EMOTIONAL INTELLIGENCE, SAMPLE EXERCISE #9: IN-CLASS ACTIVITIES TO DEVELOP NURSING STUDENT EMOTIONAL INTELLIGENCE

Specific student exercises that can be incorporated into classroom teaching include the following:

1. Class Mood/Energy check-in: Before the class arrives, on a whiteboard near the entry to the classroom, draw a large graph with "energy" on the vertical axis and "mood" on the horizontal axis. As each student arrives, they put an "x" that represents where they are on the graph. To begin the class, have a student volunteer "analyze" the data from the class.

2. Individual Mood/Energy check-in: Teaching the practice of checking in on a Mood/Energy axis is a great practice for beginning meetings with students, and for teaching them a specific practice to keep track of their feelings. Identifying where they are on the Mood/Energy graph helps them make plans for how to best manage their emotions.

3. Brain drain: Start every class by asking the class to take out a piece of paper and do "automatic writing" for 3 minutes. Automatic writing has only one rule: start and don't stop. This practice helps students "empty their emotional pockets" so they are ready to learn. At the end, have the students rip up the paper and deposit it in the trash.

4. In-class journaling: Designated time every class, even just a few minutes, for students to journal about their feelings and reactions to class material can be a great integration practice, particularly in classes that involve emotional content. This can be a requirement for the course.

REFERENCES

Codier, E. (2016). *Teaching health care in virtual space: Best practices for teaching in multi-user virtual environments.* University of Hawaii Press.

Codier, E., & Holeikaumaka, A. (2012). Virtual clinical rounds in a multi-user virtual environment (MUVE). *Journal of Nursing Education, 51*(10), 595–596. https://doi.org/10.3928/01484834-20120920-02

Codier, E., Neves, A., & Morrison, P. (2014). Teaching nursing students in a multi-user virtual environment (MUVE): A pilot study. *Annals of Nursing Practice, 1*(3), 1012.

Hutchinson, M., Hurley, J., Kozlowski, D., & Whitehair, L. (2017). The use of emotional intelligence capabilities in clinical reasoning and decision-making: A qualitative, exploratory study. *Journal of Clinical Nursing, 27*(3–4), e600-e610. https://doi.org/10.1111/jocn.14106

Kotsou, I., Mikolajczak, M., Hereen, A., Gregoire, J., & Leys, D. (2018). Improving emotional intelligence: A systematic review of existing work and future challenges. *Emotion Review, 11*(2), 151–165. https://doi.org/10.1177/1754073917735902

MacCann, C., Jiang, Y., Brown, L. E. R., Double, K. S., Bucich, M., & Minbashian, A. (2019). Emotional intelligence predicts academic performance: A meta-analysis. *Psychological Bulletin, 146*(2), 150–186. https://doi.org/10.1037/bul0000219

Mayer, J. D., Caruso, D., & Salovey, P. (1999). Emotional intelligence meets traditional standards for an intelligence. *Intelligence, 27,* 267–298. https://doi.org/10.1016/S0160-2896(99)00016-1

Rankin, B. (2013). Emotional intelligence: Enhancing values-based practice and compassionate care in nursing. *Journal of Advanced Nursing, 69*(12), 2717–2725. https://doi.org/10.1111/jan.12161

Rode, J., & Brown, K. (2019). Emotional intelligence relates to NCLEX and standardized readiness test: A pilot study. *Nurse Educator, 44*(3), 154–158. https://doi.org/10.1097/NNE.0000000000000565

Rogers, M. E. (1961). *Educational revolution in nursing.* Macmillan Publishers.

Sutton, J. (2006). Distributed cognition: Domains and dimensions. *Pragmatics and Cognition, 14*(2), 235–247. https://doi.org/10.1075/pc.14.2.05sut

10

Emotional Intelligence Across the Professional Lifespan

INTRODUCTION

In this chapter, the four (EI) abilities, identifying, understanding, using and managing emotions are applied to nurses' professional lifespan (Mayer et al., 1999). Their usual order is adapted to best align with the nursing process.

NURSING NOVICE TO EXPERT

EI Ability and the Benner Model

Research findings across many disciplines, including nursing, have demonstrated the relationship between emotional intelligence (EI) ability and job performance (see Chapter 15 for a research summary). At each level of nurse performance, from novice to expert, EI abilities support evolving performance. Interpersonal and team abilities required in advanced stages, such as leadership, conflict management, and organizational change, similarly correlate with EI ability.

Story: Yell Just A Little (From a Nurse Leader Exercise Applying Experience to EI Theory)

I love nursing, and I think nurses are just the greatest people. My career has been so satisfying, in part because I get to hang around with these great people whose work I admire so much. In some ways, this was why I made a good nurse manager. My approach was collegial, supportive, and always focused on coaching and teaching. When there were performance issues or necessary confrontations with staff, it always had a coaching, positive tone. This was fundamental to my awareness of myself as a leader, and only grew as I matured as a leader.

However, there came a time when this approach just did not work. One of my staff was a capable but profoundly irritating nurse. She was loud, brash, and unhelpful. On our busy unit, she was disruptive. I received many complaints, as she was not a team player. The staff kept telling me, "You have to yell at her," but I could not imagine that being either possible or desirable. Looking back across a long management career, I laugh at how many times I was wrong about something when my staff was right. I wondered, what if they are right? I learned to trust that group wisdom. I did not know about EI at the time, but knowing about it now, I understand how EI abilities helped me through this difficult situation.

Applying EI

Using EI: Identifying Emotions

I was confronted with disruptive behavior that did not respond to feedback. I had assumed this nurse was uncaring and disrespectful of authority, but I also had to acknowledge that something about this situation was not adding up. At the bedside, her gentleness and caring with patients made her seem like a different person. Additionally, my leadership really worked for that unit—except for her. So, what if she was not in fact, feeling what I thought she was?

Using EI: Understanding Emotions and Using Emotions to Reason ("Think/Feel")

When emotional situations don't "add up," it is a red flag. This mental disconnect often results from incorrect assumptions. Understanding this, I reevaluated the situation. When emotions are used to reason, we "think/feel," combining data from our emotional experience with data from our cognitive experience. With this troublesome nurse, the result of a think/feel process gave me several ideas. I accepted the possibility my assessment of this staff nurse's feelings may have been inaccurate, so I also stopped blaming her and acknowledged my feedback was not working. Further, I explored my staff's recommendation. Why did they want me to yell at her? Under what conditions would a raised voice be exactly what is needed?

It hit me like a lightning bolt. This nurse had grown up and lived most of her professional life in a patriarchal culture where animated exchanges, particularly about things of importance, often transpired in loud tones of voice. A loud voice indicated something was very important. In my own culture, the opposite was true. Growing up, the more important the issue, the more hushed the tone of voice. Not so for my employee. That was what my staff had been trying to make me understand. The nurse simply could not "hear" my feedback.

Using EI: Managing Emotions

I had to manage my own emotions differently. I needed to give feedback in a way this nurse could, literally, hear. I had to speak to this nurse in a firm, loud, authoritarian voice. I hated the idea. I was not sure I could do it, but I couldn't see any other way.

I practiced again and again, right up to the hour of the appointment. The nurse came to my office. I said my planned three short sentence statement about her behavior that ended with, "*and it must stop!*" I was not yelling, but I was certainly loud. My voice was stern and I punctuated the last word with a slap of my hand on my thigh.

The nurse looked at me, startled. Her eyes opened wide, but she regarded me as if she had not seen me before. She simply said, "Oh! *Okay, I get it.*" We went on to a topic she had wanted to talk about, a minor vacation issue, in our normal tones of voice, as if the first part of our appointment hadn't happened.

Story Reflection

Although incredibly uncomfortable for me, I had found a way to be heard. The nurse's behavior changed and the staff breathed a collective sigh of relief. Although I didn't know about EI abilities at the time, in retrospect they made all the difference. What was escalating into a crisis in our unit took only basic EI ability to change the outcome. It was not complicated. It did not take a disciplinary action, a consultant, or a major intervention. We did not lose a valuable employee and team member. The unit did not become defensive or toxic and I learned a difficult lesson about communication, leadership, and emotional assumptions about other people. Identifying emotions correctly, understanding them, using them to think about the situation, and managing emotions in this difficult situation made it possible to change the situation successfully.

EI APPLIED TO NURSE CAREER DEVELOPMENT

Using the Benner Model in Career Development

Benner's model of clinical proficiency is useful for understanding how a nurse learns nursing, growing from novice through levels of expertise and experience to proficiency and expert practice. EI abilities support the developmental tasks needed to achieve each level and the developing skills that help nurses' transition from one level to the next. This is particularly evident when EI is applied to interpersonal, team, conflict, and critical thinking skills. The model is less helpful for understanding career development over the whole trajectory of a nurse's professional life. Most nurses achieve proficient or expert levels of practice long before their career is over. To better explore how EI ability supports the entirety of a professional life span, a model from outside nursing is helpful.

Introduction to the Super Model

Nursing is often not simply a career choice, but a chance to integrate personal values into a career choice. Multidisciplinary research provides evidence that such integration of personal values and career choices correlates with higher levels of life and career satisfaction. Donald Super's Model of Career Development reflects this by integrating professional, personal, and developmental elements into career choice. Super's model has several elements that apply particularly well to nursing. In all the stages that Super describes, EI abilities foster both tasks inherent to individual stages and to the work necessary to transition to subsequent stages (Super et al., 1996).

Growth Stage (Imagination and Skill Preparation)

Super's first stage, Growth, begins long before an actual career choice. The Growth stage is fueled by fantasy (imagining a career), interests, and curiosity. Adults experience this stage as they envision a new career or make major career changes. They may be starting over in a totally new job, role, or work context, for which new skills, attitudes, interests, and social abilities must be developed. This happens when nursing is chosen by adults as a midlife career change.

Developmental career tasks in this stage include:

1. Shift of focus from the present to the future.
2. Increased control over life choices.
3. Self-motivation for both education and job training.
4. Self-management in work/study habits and attitudes (Super et al., 1996).

EI Ability in the Growth Stage

Nurses in the Growth stage may need new self-skills, interpersonal, group, team, or organizational skills when they change professional roles.

A former hedge fund manager who began nursing school at 40 attested to this! Research evidence demonstrates the role of EI ability in interpersonal and intrapersonal skills, effective communication, emotional problem-solving, and self-care within complex organizations.

One specific example of using EI ability in the Growth stage is managing fear, a natural part of the growth cycle. Beginning to focus on the future and trying something new and making a major life change can be scary. Understanding fear and learning to "think through it," as well as making a plan for managing fear is important for success in the Growth stage. It may make the difference between being paralyzed by fear and being able to move forward.

Exploration (Education and Preparation)

Exploration of a new career is characterized by (1) choice of career, (2) specific plans and goals, and (3) completion of education required for the career and -being hired at a first job. Future nurses in this stage take prerequisite courses required for nursing school and become nurses' aides or volunteer in a community care or hospital setting. By the end of this stage, nurses have completed nursing school and the first two stages of Benner's clinical development. For adult nurses, making career changes such as a change in role, clinical specialty, or professional context (from a hospital setting to rural public health, for example), the same stage characteristics and developmental goals apply. Education necessary for the new career is been completed, an entry-level job achieved, and initial proficiency developed (Super et al., 1996).

EI Ability in the Exploration Stage
The developmental tasks of the Exploration stage, corresponding roughly to Benner's Novice/Advanced Beginner, are daunting. Young people often leave home during this stage and experience new kinds of relationships, including collegial relationships. They begin academic programs such as nursing school, which require achievement of new individual, group, and clinical skills. In challenging programs like nursing school, identification, understanding, and management of stress become very important. Achievement of this stage's developmental goals requires acute and persistent self-awareness, self-evaluation, and self-management, as well as good relationships with peers, coworkers, mentors, and academic faculty. Nursing research (see Chapter 15) provides evidence for the role of EI in self-efficacy, relationship effectiveness, interpersonal communication, stress management, resilience, and academic achievement. EI abilities clearly correlate with the three most important elements of nursing school—scholastic achievement, clinical

performance, and nursing program completion—which makes them particularly important in this stage.

Establishment Stage (Frustration, Consolidating Skills, Increasing Responsibility)

The Establishment stage is a long period that begins as the first job in a career that stabilizes, evolves, and often changes with career opportunities and new interests. Themes in this stage include stabilizing, dealing with frustration, consolidating skills, and taking on new responsibilities.
Developmental tasks of this stage include:

1. Adapting to an organization and achieving basic competency.
2. Developing mature work habits: productivity, positive work attitudes, coworker and team relationships.
3. Taking on new levels of responsibility.

This stage corresponds to Benner's Proficiency stage. For some nurses, it corresponds to the Expert stage as well. For others, the Proficiency Stage may be their highest level of career performance (Super et al., 1996).

EI Ability in the Establishment Stage

Performance in the Establishment stage, and completion of its developmental tasks, depends largely on EI abilities. Frustration generated from organizational complexity or dysfunction, obstacles to important goals, or thwarting of personal achievements can challenge adults in this stage. Adapting to changing organizational goals, managing conflicts between career and family life, and gaining increased levels of responsibility all require identification of emotions, understanding emotions, reasoning with them, and self-management. The body of nursing EI research reflects this. EI abilities correlate with constructive adaptation to change, positive approaches to conflict, successful teamwork, communication effectiveness, and prosocial organizational behaviors.

The transition from the Establishment stage (Super et al., 1996) to the next stage is rigorous for nurses and the need for EI abilities is particularly acute. The transition from Proficiency to Expert (Benner, 1984) most often requires expanding clinical practice and formalizing leadership and/or mentoring responsibilities. In this stage, nurses are often required to float to other clinical areas, increasing their clinical skills and adapting to different teams and clinical environments. New leadership responsibilities often take the form of charge nurse duties, and orienting new employees similarly requires formal mentoring responsibilities. Participation in hospital committees may be required. For nurses new to these roles, the frustrations ubiquitous to working with groups and organizations are often challenging. The new interpersonal and organizational skills required are not always mastered. Some nurses, even after many years of practice, may not have clinical, leadership, or mentoring abilities necessary to advance to this level.

Maintenance Stage (Holding, Updating, Stagnation, and Innovating)

In Super's Maintenance stage, a steady state has developed in the career. Themes of this stage have to do with requisite updating and innovating of skills as the work environment changes. Stagnation can occur without innovation and updating of skills. Nurses in stagnation, who have difficulty with new equipment, procedures, patient populations, or organizational goals, may begin to exhibit significant performance issues (Super et al., 1996).

EI Ability in the Maintenance Stage

In this stage, two trajectories are common: stagnation and adaptation, and EI abilities may determine which occurs. If a nurse can successfully negotiate changes on the unit, be aware of their feelings and those of others, understand their feelings within the context of the change, and think/feel their way to a plan for adaptation, the nurse may adapt effectively to change. If these skills are not used, change resistance behaviors can arise resulting in both stagnated performance and sometimes a vicious cycle of negative feedback and negative performance reviews. Managing such employees can be challenging. Coaching these nurses to improve their EI abilities may be useful.

Disengagement Stage (Decelerating, Retirement Planning, Career Exit, and Retirement Living)

Super describes Disengagement as the final stage of a career. Themes enumerated for this stage include slowing down, decelerating, retirement planning, and transition into retirement. The developmental goal of this stage is an exit from the career. In most disciplines, the gradual transition to retirement is often accompanied by adjustments in job expectations and focus. Deceleration of job responsibilities is expected.

This stage is often different for nurses. In nursing roles, a deceleration of job responsibilities may not be practical. A clinical nurse at the bedside the day before they retire is expected to meet the same performance standards as any other nurse. A nurse manager typically works fully up until their day of departure. There also is an ethos in nursing that "once a nurse, always a nurse." Retired people usually refer to their professional identities in the past tense, "I was a teacher," "I was a firefighter." But how often do you hear "I was a nurse?" Because of their propensity for integrating personal values fully into their professional identity, nurses commonly fuse their personal and professional identities, and even when not actively working after retirement, this often persists within the nurse's self-concept. Nurses also often work beyond 65 and many who fully retire still maintain active nursing licenses. Even when fully disengaged from the nursing workforce, many retired nurses use their nursing skills in volunteer activities. This complicates the developmental tasks of the Disengagement stage.

EI ABILITY IN THE DISENGAGEMENT STAGE

Navigation of this last stage of a nurse's career requires effective self-reflection and self-management, as well as navigation of closure, grieving, and relationship transitions. These are difficult challenges complicated by fusing of personal/professional identity. Collegial relationships in this stage provide support, feedback, reflection, and emotional self-management. Because of the important role of EI in effective communication, interpersonal relationships, and personal emotional wellness, these abilities are crucial for effectively navigating the Disengagement stage.

Applying Nurse EI to Developmental Phenomenology

Most career models prior to Super focused on career choice as a "one-shot" decision. The goal of these models was mostly to assist people in matching their characteristics and interests with a corresponding career. This matching determined the choice of a person's career which, short of making changes mid-career, was the biggest determinant of career trajectory. In contrast, Super described development of a life-long career as the consequence of a series of career choices. Within career stages, he also described "sub-cycles" in which an expert makes a career change that renders them a novice again. This is common among nurses, who have a wide range of options for specialty, role, and clinical contexts under the umbrella of professional nursing. An ICU nurse might leave the hospital to find satisfaction in home care or hospice. An expert clinical nurse could become a nurse educator or CNS. Access to these choices across life span offers nurses many options to reduce stress, adapt their career to support other elements of their life, increase job satisfaction, develop new interests, and experience continuous learning as they grow and change.

For nurses with extensive sub-cycle experience, the learning curve for each cycle may grow shorter. At the start of a sub-cycle, some aspects of the nurse's practice revert to the Novice/Advanced Beginner stage (Table 10.1). For example, a clinical nurse takes an advanced practice role after completing a master's degree in business. Because other aspects of their practice, such as basic clinical, group, team, and organizational skills are usually already at a Proficient/Expert level, this expert clinical nurse may progress through a sub-cycle and progress quickly to expert leader. Nurses who thrive on change may have many such sub-cycles across their career and with experience, shorten the duration of sub-cycle achievement. Life-long learning, which represents sub-cycling on a micro level, may also be supported by EI ability.

TABLE 10.1 Example of Career Decisions Across One Nurse's Professional Life Span

SAMPLE CAREER REFLECTIONS	SUPER'S MODEL	BENNER'S MODEL OF CLINICAL COMPETENCY
"I always wanted to be a nurse, so I worked hard in high school to keep my grades up and I volunteered at a local nursing home."	Stage: Growth (Imagination, interest)	Novice
"I got interested in cardiac nursing in nursing school."	Stage: Growth (Development of interests) shifting to Exploration (Trying out roles, tentative choices)	Novice
"Cardiac care was my first job as a new graduate."	Establishment (Entry-level skill building)	Novice/Advanced Beginner transition to Competent
"After a few years, I enjoyed being charge nurse."	Shift back to Exploration (Change of roles)	May revert to Advanced Beginner
"I needed a challenge so I transferred to cardiac ICU."	Change of setting and specialty focus (ICU); Exploration shifting rapidly to Establishment	Proficient
"I wanted to develop my leadership skills, so I was promoted to nurse manager."	Exploration shifting rapidly to Establishment (Change of role and position within the organization)	Return to previous level for sub-cycling, then Proficient, for some nurses, Expert

(continued)

TABLE 10.1 Example of Career Decisions Across One Nurse's Professional Lifespan (*Continued*)

SAMPLE CAREER REFLECTIONS	SUPER'S MODEL	BENNER'S MODEL OF CLINICAL COMPETENCY
"I started to burn out, so I moved to the cardiac rehab unit in a large business complex."	Change of setting	Novice; typically moves through following stages more quickly than the first time. May advance beyond previous cycle's highest level of proficiency
"I had always loved teaching, and needed a day job while my kids were little, so I applied for a clinical instructor position at a community college."	Change of role, change in specialty, change in setting	Novice; typically moves through following stages more quickly than the first time. May advance beyond previous cycle's highest level of proficiency
"I really needed a total change. After my divorce, I was a flight nurse and went all over the world transporting patients."	Change of role, change in specialty, change in setting	Novice; typically moves through following stages more quickly than the first time. May advance beyond previous cycle's highest level of proficiency
"After retirement, I worked with the local Red Cross for medical response in the event of a disaster."	Change in specialty, role, setting	Variable

DEVELOPING EMOTIONAL INTELLIGENCE ABILITY

SAMPLE EMOTIONAL INTELLIGENCE DEVELOPMENT EXERCISE #10: FRUSTRATION MANAGEMENT: LEAKING AND THRESHOLDS

In the management of a career across a lifespan, two of the greatest challenges are energy management and management of challenging emotions. The EI abilities of identification of emotions and understanding emotions are especially helpful with both these challenges.

1. Energy management: Leaking: *"Are you leaking?"* When strong emotions are in play, particularly negative emotions, it is very easy to "leak" energy by pouring energy into these emotions. For example, on one very challenging clinical unit, whose fast pace

and constantly changing environment was particularly demanding, a common phrase was used, "Are you leaking?" This question was usually asked in a funny way, but the point was obvious. "I know you are feeling very (whatever the emotion is), but can you really afford to pour energy into it right now?"

2. Threshold management: Emotionally healthy and resilient people have high thresholds for negative emotions. It takes a lot of stimulus to get them angry, frustrated, anxious, or upset. But there are lots of things that can affect those thresholds. Fatigue is a good example. When someone is really tired, or overworked, or distracted, or in pain their thresholds *drop*. So it takes much less stimuli for them to get angry, frustrated, anxious, or upset. Identifying changes in thresholds can really help a person think about and manage difficult emotions. "I am going to ask you to bear with me today. I am exhausted and my thresholds are shot! If I get frustrated easily, please understand." This is especially important in self-management of very strong emotions. Noticing when a strong emotion seems to be overtaking you, it is a good idea to check your thresholds.The strength of the emotion might have resulted from a drop in your usual threshold.

REFERENCES

Benner, P. (1984). *From novice to expert: Excellence and power in clinical nursing practice.* Addison-Wesley.

Mayer, J. D., Caruso, D., & Salovey, P. (1999). Emotional intelligence meets traditional standards for an intelligence. *Intelligence, 27,* 267–298. https://doi.org/10.1016/S0160-2896(99)00016-1

Super, D. E., Savickas, M. L., & Super, C. M. (1996). The life-span, life-space approach to careers. In D. Brown, L. Brooks, & Associates (Eds.), *Career choice and development* (3rd ed., pp. 121–178). Jossey-Bass.

11

Emotional Intelligence, Nurse Leadership, and Organizational Change

INTRODUCTION

Emotional intelligence (EI) is defined as the "ability to recognize the meanings of emotions .... and to reason and problem-solve on the basis of them" (Mayer et al., 1999, p. 267). In this chapter EI is operationalized with the following skills:

1. Accurate identification of emotions in self and others
*2. Understanding emotions
*3. Using emotions to reason (integrating thinking and feeling), and
4. Managing emotions.
(Mayer et al., 1999).

For the purposes of this text, skills 2 and 3 are reversed from the published Mayer et al. order. This is done to better align the four abilities with the nursing process illustrated throughout this text.

This chapter examines nurse leader (EI) abilities specifically as they apply to organizational change. This chapter illustrates use of EI abilities as they enhance the following leader skills: managing clinical outcomes, change resistance, supervisory relationships, team conflict and consensus-building, and managing time.

NURSE LEADERSHIP AND EMOTIONAL INTELLIGENCE (EI)

More than twenty years of international research across dozens of disciplines and hundreds of research studies has provided ample evidence that EI correlates with leader effectiveness, wellness, and career longevity. Nursing EI research has built on these findings and validated them, supporting the importance of EI for nurse leaders (see research summary, Chapter 15). Nurse leaders can and must utilize EI skills to face the unprecedented challenges confronting them daily within the context of a rapidly changing industry. These skills are among the most important for facilitating organizational change. For that reason, this chapter focuses on change skills including the following: management of clinical outcomes, change resistance, supervisory relationships, team conflict, consensus processes, and leader self-care.

APPLYING EI ABILITIES IN MANAGEMENT OF ORGANIZATIONAL OUTCOMES

Optimizing organizational outcomes invariably involves change processes. Continuous quality improvement, employee performance evaluation, and process changes necessitated by new clinical procedures all work together to create an environment where change is the status quo. Nurse leaders must develop abilities that support themselves, their staff, and the organization in this constantly dynamic industry. An early meta-analysis of 141 EI leadership research studies across all disciplines provided evidence for a relationship between EI and positive leadership outcomes (Mills, 2009). In some of the earliest nurse EI research, EI significantly correlated with important organizational outcomes such as customer satisfaction, fiscal outcomes, and organizational resilience amid change (Cummings et al., 2005). Meta-analysis of nurse leader EI research concluded EI is a useful tool for nurse managers, particularly as it is related to effective leadership outcomes that support successful navigation of change (Akerjordet & Severinsson, 2018; Prezerakos, 2018).

The skills necessary for leaders to navigate change successfully all correlate with EI ability. The EI abilities enable leaders to manage themselves, their staff, and organizations through the challenging emotional topography of change processes that are required to improve organizational outcomes. This is especially evident in one of a nurse manager's most difficult challenges: managing resistance to change.

Using EI Abilities in Change Resistance

Change resistance is an intrinsic part of the change process. It is not a sign that the change process is ineffective. What is of concern is resistance that begins to obstruct change, or when change resistance interferes with performance, teamwork, or safety. Table 11.1 lists common manifestations of resistance to change, their symptoms, and common negative outcomes.

TABLE 11.1 Change Resistance: Symptoms and Negative Outcomes

RESISTANCE SYMPTOM	SYMPTOMS	NEGATIVE OUTCOMES
Emotions	Negative emotions, self-centered orientation	Contagion of negativity, reduced interpersonal effectiveness, increased conflict, reduced customer satisfaction
Disengagement	Avoidance, reduced communication, apathy, low morale	Poor performance, team dysfunction, reduced customer satisfaction
Performance	Poor quality and quantity of work, noncompliance, increased medical errors, under-involvement in change process	Financial loss, reduced customer satisfaction, miscommunication, team dysfunction, noncompliance, compromised patient safety
Disruptive behavior	Inappropriate behavior, bullying, conflict, undermining and passive/aggressive actions, increased involvement in change process but in a disruptive way	Miscommunication and team dysfunction, team/energy lost in personnel action
Negativity	Intentional miscommunication (rumors, gossip), focusing on negative outcomes, celebrating failure, overt negativity about change process	Contagion of negativity, reduced interpersonal effectiveness, increased conflict, reduced customer satisfaction
Avoidance	Reinforcing old behaviors, avoiding the change, working around the new requirements to revert to the old, refuse responsibility	Loss of accountability and informal leadership, parallel processes as new and old coexist, covert threat to change process
Creation of barriers	Cadre of those opposed to change formed, participation solicited	Mistrust, secrecy, paranoia, splitting in team goals, recruitment to threaten change process
Controlling behavior	Overt undermining of change process, advocating for return to the old way	Overt threat to success of change process

Source: Changing Minds. (n.d.). Signs of resistance. http://changingminds.org/disciplines/change_management/resistance_change/sign_resistance.htm

Any one of the resistance elements listed above has enough power to effectively derail a change process, particularly once a culture of resistance is established. When resistant staff recruit others, subsequent team splitting undermines change as well as staff morale, performance, and interpersonal relationships. This resistance manifests interpersonally with subtle pressure and overt bullying. All negative elements of change resistance can be effectively addressed with EI abilities. For example, a leader could (1) identify emotions such as anger or frustration from the change, (2) teach about change resistance to facilitate understanding of the emotions related to this process, (3) model "think/feel" management of bullying behavior, and (4) model emotionally problem-solving by making plans for emotional self-management and group management during stressful change. These actions can prevent resistance from progressing from a maladaptive response by individual staff members to a culture of resistance that effectively undermines the desired change.

Story: Unchanged

The hospital made a major commitment to improve patient safety. A consultant had been hired, meetings held, buy-in of senior leaders achieved, planning for long-range and short-range strategy completed, and education of the staff had begun. At every step of the process, the administration made significant effort to include clinical staff in revising procedures. The proposed change involved three major elements of nursing shift change report:

1. The shift change report would relocate to the patient's bedside, so IVs and equipment could be checked by both shifts.
2. The format of shift change report would standardize all elements required for reporting, including safety concerns and risk factors.
3. Patients would be included in report, and goals for each shift which would be summarized on a whiteboard at each patient's bedside.

This change was never presented as optional. Medical error data had been presented to the group that clearly indicated changes were necessary. In the beginning, resistance was subtle. Resistant staff grumbled, "The patient should not be able to hear what we say in report." Because the change was under the banner of patient safety, the staff refrained from overt complaints, but "didn't like" the shift change format. Comments such as, "I have my own way of keeping everything organized so I don't forget anything" surfaced. Because bedside shift report was not recorded, the implementation team could not monitor either location compliance or shift report content compliance unless a member was physically present.

As the staff accommodated to the change, intensive monitoring took place for weeks.

The first overt resistance behaviors were verbal negativity, grudging compliance, and splitting of the staff. The staff was forming into two camps: those who changed and those who did not. Although shift report had moved out of the old shift report lounge, it began moving further and further from patient bedsides. It started at corridors outside patients' rooms, then onto corridor furniture, and finally to family rest areas at the end of hallways. In this manner, the location of the shift report, one of the important aspects of the change, was totally subverted. Other aspects of the change were undermined. The whiteboard plans of care for each patient were similarly undermined. At first, they were not kept up-to-date, and eventually not used all. Insidiously, the unit old-timers pressured newer staff to revert to the old ways. Eventually, unless a change process monitor was physically present, very little bedside shift reporting was done at all. The standardized shift report content was almost completely abandoned as staff reverted back to their own preferred means of giving report.

Applying EI

How could this story, typical of change resistance, have been different? Research evidence demonstrates that leader EI abilities result in nurses more effectively navigating organizational change (Cummings et al., 2005). These abilities can also address and mitigate change resistance. The intentional use of EI abilities could have changed the trajectory of the change process, as well as the degree to which resistance was successful. Change makes all of us uncomfortable, that is natural, but the only way to make our patients safer is to be willing to change.

Using EI to Manage Change Resistance: Identifying Emotions

What if the nurse leaders had done staff education on change resistance? Teaching staff about typical emotional responses to change, even posting the resistance chart on the unit, might have made identifying emotional resistance and the negative behaviors associated with it easier. "You might start hearing people say negative things about this change. Remember, the goal is to make patients safer!" Also, teaching staff to identify change resistance recruitment is very important. "You might feel pressure from people who don't want to make the change. Pay attention if you start to feel pressured or bullied!" Identifying resistance emotions and resistance symptoms publicly and explicitly keeps resistance from taking root and progressing. Talking about them openly during performance reviews is also helpful.

Using EI Abilities to Manage Change Resistance: Understanding Emotions

After identifying resistance emotions and behaviors, understanding them is an important next step. For example, some of the emotional negativity stemmed from fear. Everyone knew many of the older staff, who had a lot of informal power, gave poor reports. Newer staff found confronting this problem awkward since it had been tolerated for years. Accountability had never been successfully addressed.

Using EI to Manage Change Resistance: Using Emotions to Reason and Managing Emotions

Providing unit education ahead of time could have decreased resistance behaviors and given the staff language to talk about it when pressure and bullying surfaced. A unit party to celebrate the first few weeks of the change, where staff could socialize and emphasize positive progress, is one simple solution. Identifying emotions, understanding them, and using them to think about both the change process and resistance could have enabled the nurse manager to select interventions to address the emotional issues underlying the noncompliance instead of focusing on the noncompliance as the problem.

While dealing with resistance meant addressing fear ("Doing things differently can be scary. Let's be patient with each other as we get used to the new shift report"), it also meant addressing the loss of social time in the breakroom before shift report. With bedside reports, the oncoming shift didn't have a chance to relax together and check-in before the shift began. Understanding this emotional need could have improved compliance and reduced resistance behaviors.

APPLYING EI TO TEAM PROCESS MANAGEMENT

Effective leaders are masters at working with teams, and nurse leaders are especially so. Their management of nurse, administrative and interdisciplinary teams are among their most important, challenging, and rewarding tasks. Consensus building and conflict management are among the most important team processes that nurse leaders must cultivate. For both, EI abilities play a crucial role.

Applying EI to Group Consensus

Using EI ability helps nurse leaders to manage groups and teams more effectively. Much of leaders' work is in groups of all sizes, so the

EXHIBIT 11.1 Using EI Abilities in Consensus

PHASES OF CONSENSUS PROCESS	RELEVANT EMOTIONAL INTELLIGENCE ABILITIES
Phase 1: Brainstorming ideas for problem solution	Identifying emotions correctly in self and others, Understanding emotions
Phase 2: Identifying common themes	Understanding emotions, Using emotions to reason
Phase 3: Formulating priorities among themes	Identifying emotions correctly in self and others, Understanding emotions, Using emotions to reason, Managing emotions in self and others

Source: Mayer, J. D., Caruso, D., & Salovey, P. (1999). Emotional intelligence meets traditional standards for an intelligence. *Intelligence, 27,* 267–298. https://doi.org/10.1016/S0160-2896(99)00016-1

development of team management skills enhances leader effectiveness. An example of this is the use of EI leader ability in guiding the consensus process. Across all the phases of consensus development, EI ability can be used to both guide and enhance the process.

For nursing and interdisciplinary teams to function effectively, leaders need skills in consensus building. Performance of this skill is rarely taught, evaluated, or developed in either nursing school or graduate-level nurse leader education. As illustrated in Exhibit 11.1, EI abilities contribute specifically to the three main phases of the consensus process.

Using EI Abilities: Consensus Phase I

In the first phase of group consensus, the group brainstorms ideas about issues and possible solutions. In a clinical setting, this could include anything from issues that impact a problem, such as interpersonal or group dynamics, organizational issues such as short staffing or miscommunication, or even clinical issues such as interdisciplinary team conflict. The rule in this phase is "no editing, judging, or prioritizing" and the goal is to get as many issues/solutions on the table as possible.

Identifying emotions and understanding emotions in oneself and others is crucial during this phase. For example, if one staff member has a strong emotional reaction to someone else's contribution ("I hate that idea, it will never work!"), identifying and recognizing the strength of that emotion enables the staff member to use what they understand about emotions and consensus ("Wait, sorry, this is only Phase I! No editing yet! I can raise my concerns later."). Many items on the brainstorm list never get to Phase II. If staff spend emotional energy and interpersonal goodwill on a disagreement during Phase I, both may have been wasted on an idea that wasn't even going to make it to the next stage. Understanding emotions also helps maintain personal communication discipline at this stage. Brainstorming only works effectively under the "no editing, judging, or prioritizing" rule.

Using EI Abilities: Consensus Phase II

In the second phase of consensus, the group identifies themes among the brainstormed items from Phase I. All four of the EI abilities support this complex phase while the brainstormed items are categorized and prioritized. Identifying emotions correctly, both in oneself and others, can help clarify this process. Understanding emotions like defensiveness can prevent derailing the consensus. When a group is problem-solving, defensive feelings can arise if people feel judged or undervalued. Defensiveness is a highly charged emotion that can hijack a discussion easily and distract from the group task. However, it often responds well to acknowledgment, especially public acknowledgment. For example, "Jack, everyone knows how hard you have worked on this, and no one is criticizing that. We are just all trying to find some new ways to get our budget under control." By identifying and acknowledging Jack's defensiveness, the consensus process is not derailed by it, and Jack can stay actively engaged.

Using EI Abilities: Consensus Phase III

Identifying, understanding, using, and managing emotions can help a leader through the third consensus phase, which culminates in the selection of a few summary or action items. Disappointment, for example, may arise when brainstormed items are not included on the list. When the leader identifies this, they prevent disappointed group members from dropping out of the consensus process. "I am really disappointed that my idea didn't make the list, but maybe we can come back to it another time. For now, I am ready to move on." Modeling disappointment like this supports the group decision and models moving on. It also signals to the group that the idea may come up again in the future.

Applying EI to Conflict Management

As summarized in Chapter 15, there is ample evidence from multidisciplinary research that EI ability is associated with positive conflict skills for individuals and within teams. Using EI ability in conflict interactions changes interpersonal power dynamics and can result in stronger relationships and more collaboration within the change process. An illustration from the martial art aikido makes this clear.

When two traditional martial artists are joined in an attack, one force meets another force and the stronger, faster, or more agile person "wins." This is the traditional model of conflict resolution. For example, a nurse leader wants a change in the unit, they have the power, so they "make" the staff comply. One force (the leader) confronts another force (the staff). The leader has more power, so the staff is forced to comply with the will of the leader.

What is an alternative? In aikido, when faced with an attack, the person "attacked" quickly and smoothly moves out of the way, lining up with the attacker. The person attacked has literally physically lined up with their attacker. Instead of "my way versus your way," it is as if the attacker says, "let me see from your perspective." In EI terms, the person attacked is willing to get off their own position and idea long enough to see things from the other person's perspective. From this position, they can more accurately identify the emotions of the other person. By getting off their own "position" for a moment, the "win/lose and who is stronger?" approach to the conflict has changed dramatically. Instead of "stronger versus weaker and winning versus losing," the goal becomes shared understanding. In a very physical way, emotional perspective is identified, understanding achieved, thinking about the situation has shifted, and a different solution other than simply overpowering the other person is achieved.

Story Reflection: Unchanged

In the story about shift report, if the nurse leader had used the traditional, "who has the most power," approach to conflict resolution, she might have said, "You will do report at the bedside because I have the power to make you. If you keep doing it in the report room, I will use disciplinary action." Using EI abilities and the aikido approach, the leader might instead say, "Oh! You miss having time with your shift peers before starting the shift. Let's do a 5-minute shift overview in the report room with everyone present, then go to the bedside for detailed reports." By abandoning the traditional power position for a moment, the leader can think/feel with new information and hypothesize that the resistance could have originated from the emotional and social loss of a small group huddle at the beginning of a shift or from fear of failing to give an improved report. The leader can then manage the emotional situation differently and propose a new solution. Using the aikido model, the nurse manager in this scenario is willing to get off their own position long enough to "see" where the staff is coming from and suggest a solution that addresses the staff concerns within the context of the required change. In this case, by using EI abilities in the conflict, a very different outcome is possible.

APPLYING EI TO LEADER RELATIONSHIPS

Story: The Ghost of Colleen

Sally had been a staff nurse on the unit for nearly her whole nursing career and now was a few years from retirement. She was a lovely person, supportive of her colleagues, and well-liked by her coworkers and the new nurse manager on her unit. However, her performance was always borderline. Her personnel file reflected many unsuccessful performance improvement interventions and sick leave overuse from migraine headaches. The new unit nurse manager quickly realized Sally's consistent clinical performance problems meant it would not be long before Sally's performance would need to be addressed again. Sure enough, Sally made a medication error and an appointment was scheduled to discuss it.

When Sally came to the manager's office the day of the appointment, she sat down and looked at her manager with a "deer in the headlights" look on her face. The nurse manager was experienced and had done plenty of disciplinary counseling. She was good at it, but Sally's emotional affect struck her as unusual. It was out of proportion considering the issue and not consistent with the good relationship the two had forged in the preceding months.

Applying EI Abilities

Using EI: Identifying Emotions

The nurse manager began to speak about the medication error. It was pretty cut and dry, a variation in protocol. There wasn't much interpretation involved. The nurse's frozen demeanor didn't change, and she didn't speak. Even the manager's deliberately warm and nonjudgmental approach was not getting through. A bit frustrated, the nurse manager asked, "Has this kind of mistake happened before?"

Sally was suddenly energized and animated. Just about in tears, she said, "Oh, yes, I have been in this horrible little room many, many times."

The nurse manager was taken aback at her intense and highly emotional response. Following "a hunch," she changed the subject and asked about Sally's relationship with her prior supervisor, Colleen.

Then tears spilled over. Sally described being terrified by her supervisor, by the threats of firing. She talked about how afraid she had been. She reported being constantly fearful that she would lose her job. She was afraid of being in charge on a night shift or orienting new employees because additional responsibilities meant bigger mistakes that would end her career. In her office, in "that horrible little room," the nurse manager had a terrified employee in a flashback. The positive rapport with her new manager didn't help. Sally couldn't hear her new manager's words; they were drowned out by the toxic relationship with her previous manager.

Using EI: Understanding Emotions

When levels of fear are high, physiology takes over. Fight/flight results in an adrenalin dump that widens and then narrows the visual field, creating tunnel vision. Emotional thresholds change, resulting in irritability, hyper-responsiveness, and a decreased ability to process emotions. Touch is often perceived as threatening. It is difficult to take in new information or communicate due to amygdalar hijacking. Understanding all this, the manager knew her relationship with Sally, and indeed Sally's future as a nurse, could ride on what she did next. The manager could not change Sally's past. Nor could she avoid dealing with Sally's very real performance problems. But she could address Sally's fear that was blocking everything else and creating a vicious cycle of poor performance.

Using EI: Using Emotions to Reason (Think/Feel)

When we use emotions to reason, we "think/feel." We combine the data from our emotional experience with data from our cognitive experience.

Sally was paralyzed by fear. The new manager knew she could not forge a new, more constructive relationship with Sally unless she helped Sally break the fearful pattern of the past. When the nurse manager used her understanding of emotions she identified, and used this to think differently about her employee, it made her interventions better.

Using EI: Managing Emotions

The manager told Sally the conferences with her old boss sounded awful and asked how Sally had dealt with them. Despite her tears, Sally met her manager's eye squarely and said, "I get migraines."

With that answer, the manager knew if she looked through the personnel records, she would see every conference between Sally and her supervisor was followed by a sick call. The polarized and emotionally charged relationship with her previous supervisor never addressed the performance problems, and Sally's fear gave her migraine headaches.

The nurse manager needed to get through Sally's fear. She said, "Sounds to me like we got the ghost of Colleen in this room."

Unbelievably, Sally laughed. "You got that right."

The manager got up and held the door for Sally, saying, "Let's get out of here!"

Once they were in a quiet lounge area on the unit, they sat down and finally began to talk. It was productive, it was clear, and they were on the same page. They talked through the error. The conversation ended on a positive note. Sally did not call in sick the next day.

Sally and her unit leader were not done with the ghost of Colleen. Sally continued to have performance issues, and sometimes during difficult conversations she looked tense. Her manager would raise eyebrows and ask, "Colleen?" Sally would laugh and say, "No, I'm good." Their relationship stayed strong during the required process to improve Sally's performance. Slowly, the ghost of Colleen faded. Sally was never the strongest nurse on the unit, but her positive and encouraging personality remained valuable to the unit.

Story Reflection

Only a few simple EI abilities made the difference between a traumatized employee stuck in a vicious cycle and a unit no longer disrupted by sick calls and an underperforming nurse. The relationship with Sally's unit leader stayed strong. The manager had helped Sally recover from an emotional trauma and improve her attendance and performance. The team was saved the loss of a valued member, and the quality of team care improved along with Sally's performance. This story illustrates the power of EI ability to increase the effectiveness and impact of leader relationships, whether they be relationships with employees, peers, or line relationships within an organization.

APPLYING EI TO LEADER TIME MANAGEMENT

Most nurse managers would agree with the phrase, "My time is driven not by what I can do but what I must do." Most times, management systems reflect the same, seemingly common-sense approach to time management; start with the leadership goals, then prioritize according to the most time-sensitive or those with the highest financial or safety risk. However, using EI ability to manage time starts with the opposite assumption: "My time is driven by what I can do more than what I must do." This constitutes a fundamental stress and energy management strategy in the short run and contributes to long-term thriving and burnout prevention across the trajectory of a nurse leader's career.

Story: Monday Morning

It was barely 8 a.m. on Monday morning, and the ICU nurse manager was already exhausted. She was fighting a cold and the third cup of coffee was not helping get her going. Her eye was on her earliest possible departure to home and early to bed. The schedule for her week was overbooked, the unit was very busy and there had been last-minute sick calls. What she had to do for even the next few hours seemed overwhelming. What if she worked this situation with EI, beginning with herself and what she could do? Using a simple EI tool offers an entirely different approach to "Just do it."

Applying EI Abilities

Using EI: Identifying Emotions

One important way to use EI in time management is illustrated using Figure 11.1. On this chart, the vertical axis is labeled "Energy," and the horizontal axis is labeled "Mood." This Mood/Energy chart is a fast way to assess resources at the beginning of a day, meeting, or at the beginning of work on a project. This practical example shows how to use EI to improve leadership effectiveness.

The manager started by identifying her own emotions. She had very low energy, but actually, she was in a pretty good mood. Upon reflection, she realized that she was excited about greeting a new leader who had recently joined the organization. Today was the new manager's first day.

Using EI: Understanding Emotions

The human body and human emotions are inextricably connected. The nurse manager understood the connection between her physical and emotional energy. Her moods, her emotional baseline, were connected to

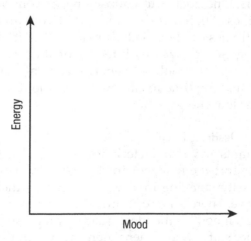

FIGURE 11.1 EI assessment: mood and energy.
Source: Original to author

her physical well-being. Both needed to be addressed, as each supported the other. She felt physically very low from the cold and mentally over-whelmed by the work, but her excitement about a new colleague was the fuel to plan the next hour of her day.

Using EI: Using Emotions to Reason

After using the Mood/Energy chart to identify where she was, the nurse manager used her understanding of mood and energy to pick her next actions. Instead of starting on the biggest or most pressing problem, she chose to increase both her energy and her mood by welcoming the new manager and making a date for coffee later in the day.

Using EI: Managing Emotions Using the Mood/Energy EI Assessment

This simple use of EI ability to jumpstart and fuel a typical Monday slump shows how to use EI in time management. Identifying where in the four quadrant Mood/Energy chart the leader is at a given moment and under-standing the physical/emotional phenomena of each quadrant can help the leader think/feel their way to efficient and effective self-management. For example, the leader in the previous example had low energy but higher mood (compared to the level of energy). This places the manager in Energy/Mood quadrant two.

Self-Management in Quadrant Two

In quadrant one, low energy is challenging. If energy-demanding activi-ties cannot be avoided, they should be approached carefully, conserving energy if possible. One goal is to choose energy conserving or energy-generating activities. High mood of quadrant two is an asset, a resource to draw on. If activities can be selected that use this, it can boost the low energy. For managers energized by interpersonal relationships, schedul-ing some relationship time could add energy. For a manager energized by a certain project, making time for it, even if it is not the highest priority, can help boost the low energy state.

Self-Management in Quadrant Three

The other quadrants have characteristics which, if identified and un-derstood, can support the manager in think/feeling (using emotions in reasoning), and self-managing in a way that makes their time manage-ment more effective. There is no "optimum" quadrant. It is easy to assume "high energy, high mood" is the ideal quadrant for leaders, but one man-ager noted that her staff avoided her when she was in that quadrant. The high energy/high mood made her come across as hyper and difficult to deal with, and the high energy made her physically restless. So she began planning activities with physical activity, such as safety surveys of the hospital that gave her a chance to walk around so later she could work on projects that needed more focus.

Self-Management in Quadrant Four

In high energy and low mood of quadrant four, how could available energy boost mood enough to be more effective for high priority activities? One manager used the example of working on the unit budget, a task she loathed. On the day this task had to be done, the manager used some of her available energy to move the project into a quiet corner of the cafeteria. Using available energy to "treat" herself to a change in location, her mood increased and she better tackled the budget project.

Self-Management in Quadrant One

The low energy and low mood of quadrant one requires self-care! It might be a good time for activities that don't require contact with other people. One nurse manager relegated hated tasks like filing or budget activities to quadrant one days, where she could lock herself in her office, listen to music she loved, and not focus on anything but those activities. She referred to her quadrant one days as "time in the cave."

Story Reflection

"Just do it" may be a short-term formula for success, but over a long professional career, it is a set up for burnout. Using EI abilities to plan and self-manage, even in something as basic as time management, is a force multiplier that can enhance leadership effectiveness. This contributes to both short-term and long-term effectiveness, thriving, and burnout prevention across the nurse leader's career.

NURSE LEADERSHIP RESEARCH

Nursing leadership was among the first topics for nursing research (Vitello-Cicciuo, 2002), and has been well-explored in both individual studies on specific features of nurse leadership and meta-analysis (Akerjordet & Severinsson, 2010; Codier et al., 2011). Built on a solid foundation of research in other disciplines, this research is among the best substantiated among the whole body of nursing EI research.

DEVELOPING EMOTIONAL INTELLIGENCE

SAMPLE EXERCISE #11: REWRITING HISTORY

Rewriting history can be a powerful way to review something that happened in the past, learn from it, and through the power of imagination, heal the parts that were painful. To do this, simply write down the story as objectively as possible. Stepping back from the story, reflect on how the four EI abilities worked for you, and in what ways you could have used them differently. Next, rewrite the story, including what could be done differently. Don't change the actions and words of other people in the story, only your own.

REFERENCES

Akerjordet, K., & Severinsson, E. (2010). The state of the science of emotional intelligence related to nursing leadership: An integrative review. *Journal of Nursing Management, 18*(4), 363–382. https://doi.org/10.1111/j.1365-2834.2010 .01087.x

Changing Minds. (n.d.). *Signs of resistance.* http://changingminds.org/disciplines/ change_management/resistance_change/sign_resistance.htm

Codier, E., Kamikawa, C., & Kooker, B. M. (2011) Developing the emotional intelligence of nurse managers. *Nursing Administration Quarterly, 235*(3), 1–7. https://doi.org/10.1097/NAQ.0b013e3182243ae3

Cummings, G., Hayduk, L., & Estabrooks, C. (2005). Mitigating the impact of hospital restructuring on nurses: The responsibility of emotionally intelligent leadership. *Nursing Research, 54*(1), 2–12. https://doi.org/10.1097/ 00006199-200501000-00002

Mayer, J. D., Caruso, D., & Salovey, P. (1999). Emotional intelligence meets traditional standards for an intelligence. *Intelligence, 27,* 267–298. https://doi .org/10.1016/S0160-2896(99)00016-1

Mills, L. B. (2009). A meta-analysis of the relationship between emotional intelligence and effective leadership. *Journal of Curriculum and Instruction, 3*(2). https://doi.org/10.3776/joci.2009.v3n2p22-38

Prezerakos, P. E. (2018). Nurse managers' emotional intelligence and effective leadership: A review of the current evidence. *Open Nursing Journal, 12*(1), 86–92. https://doi.org/10.2174/1874434601812010086

Vitello, J. (2002). Exploring emotional intelligence: Implications for nurse leaders. *Journal of Nursing Administration, 32*(4), 203–210. https://doi .org10.1097/00005110-200204000-00009

12

Emotional Intelligence and Nurse Resilience

INTRODUCTION

This chapter illustrates use of four (EI) abilities, identifying, understanding, using and managing emotions to promote nurse resilience (Mayer et al., 1999). Their usual order is adapted to best align with the nursing process. Salutogenic and relaxation response theories are incorporated to illustrate specific ways to support nurse thriving and intrapersonal, interpersonal, and team wellness.

SALUTOGENESIS

Changing the Mind: Emotional "Dis-eases" and Emotional Wellness

Medical sociologist Dr. Antonovsky was troubled. Reviewing data from a study on aging he was working on in the 1970s, he stumbled on research findings that rocked his world and changed his mind, leading to development of a theory that would change ideas about stress, wellness, and emotional health. Dr. Antonovsky's interest in aging and human emotional survival in extreme stress and punishing trauma had led him to compare the emotional health of women who had survived Nazi concentration camps with women in a control group. Nearly a third (29%) of women who had survived the camps had positive emotional health. In the "normal" control group, the figure was 51%. Why were women imprisoned in concentration camps only somewhat (20%) less emotionally healthy than the "normal" population? Instead of examining what had gone wrong in the emotional health of concentration camp survivors, he wondered why they stayed emotionally and physically healthy after even the most extreme emotional trauma. For the answer, he focused on their remarkable resilience.

Salutogenic Theory

Instead of understanding wellness as the absence of disease, he suggested that wellness was created by a set of emotional abilities. These abilities generated wellness despite trauma, stress, and emotional experiences that would be expected to cause emotional pathology. He named this idea, "salutogenesis" (Antonovsky, 1987). Antonovsky defined salutogenesis (from the Greek, "salus" or "health," and "genesis," which means "origin"), as the means by which people manage stress and stay well. His work provides a theoretical framework for a kind of emotional resiliency that prevents disease and promotes life-long emotional wellness. His salutogenic theory offers a different view of stress, burnout, and professional thriving, one in which emotional intelligence (EI) ability has a positive role (Antonovsky, 1987).

Nurse Burnout

Burnout depletes the ranks of good nurses. It causes good nurses to leave the profession, sometimes well into their career and sometimes surprisingly early after nursing school. Its effects diminish nurses' capacity to practice safely and professionally. Burnout also inhibits nurses' ability to survive the crippling emotional effects of the chronic emotional labor that is ubiquitous to nursing. A 2019 study of 2,000 nurses found 16% reported being burned out, and an additional 45% denied burnout but reported burnout symptoms such as disengagement, emotional distance from the team, diminished morale, and enough emotional distance from patients to negatively affect patient care (Nurse.org, 2020). The World Health Organization (WHO) does not label burnout as a disease but describes it as a syndrome resulting from chronic work stress, with a cluster of symptoms including loss of energy, emotional and physical exhaustion, emotional and mental distancing, and negativity (WHO, 2019). Because of its accompanying cognitive dysfunction, a variety of preventive measures, including cognitive-behavioral therapy, cognitive restructuring, and a variety of methods for stress management have been suggested for burnout prevention (Santoft et al., 2019). Treatment of established burnout has proven more difficult. The low energy and general negativity of burned-out staff works against treatment and in some cases, burnout treatment can actually decrease professional efficacy.

APPLYING EI ABILITIES TO SALUTOGENESIS AND BURNOUT PREVENTION

EI abilities operationalize a salutogenic approach to nurse burnout prevention and treatment. The identification of emotions and emotional patterns is a powerful first step.

Using EI: Identifying Emotions and the Role of Control

Identification of emotions, like perfectionism and control, that place nurses at burnout risk, may help prevent burnout. The need to feel "in control" is practically universal among professional nurses. The nursing process, the essential core of professional nursing practice, is based on the presumption that nursing assessment, diagnosis, intervention, and reassessment can control patient outcomes. Listen to nurses talk on a busy day, "I am on top of it," "I am dealing with it," "I am coping," "I just manage." Research findings show many nurses report control-focused coping mechanisms like this, even as they are aware that such approaches not only don't work but in some cases may have negative consequences (Codier et al., 2013; Martins et al., 2010).

Using EI: Understanding Emotions

Nurses need to understand emotions before they can manage them. For example, the emotional need for control is almost universally acknowledged as a positive coping mechanism, but research does not support this. Dr. Antonovsky's research concluded a sense of feeling in control was not primary or even required to be emotionally healthy. This challenged the traditional idea that effective coping requires a sense of control. His research also concluded that emotional health was not merely the absence of disease, but the presence of emotional wellness. In the salutogenic model, health is created by the combined effects of a (1) a meaning-filled life, (2) arising from that meaning, a sense that life is understandable and manageable, and (3) the "sense of coherence" this creates. What the sense of coherence is based on (world view, personal values, or religion) does not seem to matter. In the salutogenic model, wellness arises from this meaning, manageability, and coherence. For nurses, salutogenesis offers an approach to professional life that engages the meaning nursing has for them. The three salutogenic attributes play a crucial role for nurse burnout prevention and long-term professional thriving (Antonovsky, 1987).

Story: Coherence

"My professional clinical nursing career has been all about death. I worked trauma ICU, Burn ICU, Hospice, and AIDS research. I finally accepted death as part of my professional life. Looking back over a long career, whenever I wondered, 'Why did this not create overwhelming stress and emotional damage?' I thought of one specific incident.

In nursing school, I was taking care of my first cancer patient, in the end stage of treatment. We had just had the class on Kubler-Ross' theory on stages of grieving, and I was trying to figure out how this theory could help me 'move' my patient from one stage to the next in order to 'improve' his emotional condition. When I picked up a book about grieving, the pages fell open to an aerial view of a huge, old, magnificent river, winding its way through canyons and mountains. Its power and beauty filled me as I read the picture's caption: 'The river flows. Let it flow.'

I understood. It was not about trying to move the patient to the next stage. I needed to look at my patient's grieving process like that great river. The river flows. Let it flow. I didn't need to push or manipulate or try harder. The power of my nursing care was in witnessing the process, in listening, long and hard, not judging or giving advice. Progress was not measured in stages. This moment became a foundation for decades of working with grieving and dying patients. That image saved me from a whole career of high risk, wasted emotional energy. From the very beginning, it gave me a deep admiration, respect for and love of, the grieving process. Working with dying patients and their families all of the years that followed would be challenging hard work, even heart breaking sometimes. But rather than wear me down or break me, the work drove me deeper into my life and deeper into my own wisdom and strength."

Applying EI Abilities

A sense of coherence changes a person's response to stress. The nurse's early impression of grief as a powerful, organic process like that great winding river gave a sense of coherence to future work with dying patients. This not only prevented emotional and professional exhaustion, but as a salutogenic process enabled her to thrive. This nurse was able to manage stress, prevent burnout, and develop a deep well of resilience. It began with identifying grief, learning to understand it, and then integrating reason and emotions. The touchstone image of the river flowing constituted an emotional self-management vehicle that served this nurse for decades, creating not just emotional survival but emotional thriving.

Story: The Patient From Hell

Barbara was the patient from hell, all at once manipulative, demanding, irrational, combative, and disruptive. This old, emaciated, wild-haired woman illustrated every negative stereotype about end-stage COPD patients. Daily, she tormented her favorite target, a young inexperienced ICU nurse, until they were locked in power struggles over fluid restrictions, mobility, drugs, and just about every aspect of daily care. One day, to express her rage, Barbara *ate* the nurse's shift report notes, inadvertently left on a bedside table.

When she transferred to a larger hospital, the nurse thought, "I am totally burned out, and this will be a huge challenge, but at least I won't have to take care of Barbara anymore."

Several months into her new job, the nurse was assigned an admission from the emergency room. It was a patient in end-stage COPD crisis. It was Barbara. The nurse's heart sank. She had finally begun to recover from burnout, from the trauma of relentless weeks caring for this horrible patient. Hers was a primary nursing team, one which stayed with the patients they admitted for the entire hospitalization. Over the weeks that followed, power struggles resumed where they had left off. One evening, Barbara pulled her ventilator tube out with her knees. The nurse raced into Barbara's room, frightened and furious. She was greeted with Barbara shaking her fist wildly in the air yelling, "And you ... you don't say a word!"

However, the nurse did not fall into the negative feedback cycle burnout often creates. Although they would have never admitted it, the nurse and Barbara became "frenemies." Barbara continued to be her worst patient, but the nurse slowly developed grudging respect and even affection for her. Faced with the challenge of weaning her COPD patients off ventilatory dependence, she used her deep knowledge of Barbara, and the creativity and persistence their relationship offered, to be successful. After months, Barbara was finally off the ventilator.

Then came New Year's Eve. The nurse had promised Barbara they would toast the new year together. "Sure, I believe it," Barbara answered sarcastically. The nurse had gotten a doctor's order for 30cc of champagne to be administered at midnight. But an hour before their scheduled toast, one of the worst events of the nurse's professional life occurred. She administered an IV drug to her other patient in the ICU, the patient had a severe allergic reaction to the drug and suffered a cardiac arrest. Traumatized by her role in the patient's near death, the nurse froze. Other nurses had to step in and care for her patient. As her shift ended and she got ready to go home, she was not sure if she could come back the next day or even continue to be a nurse. About to walk off the unit and go home, she remembered her promise to Barbara.

Still shaken and traumatized, she clocked out. Once she was officially off duty, she poured 30cc of champagne in two plastic drug cups and went into Barbara's room. She woke Barbara and pointed to the clock.

It was midnight. Wordlessly, she gestured to the small tray she carried, with two tiny servings of champagne bubbling in the plastic medication cups. Barbara didn't say a word but drew herself up to sit with exaggerated dignity. She reached for a cup, waited for the nurse to take her own, somberly lifted her cup to toast the nurse, and then drank. The nurse did return to work the next day. She continued for a long and wonderful career, all because of Barbara and what they shared that night. Why, she was not sure, but she was sure it was true.

Applying EI Abilities

When nurses talk about dealing with burnout and other issues related to emotional labor and job stress, they usually talk in terms of programs to deal with it. They talk vaguely about self-care. Unfortunately, chronic levels of emotional labor, emotional exhaustion, physical overwork, and burnout are not easily fixed. Salutogenic theory, operationalized by EI abilities, offers a different approach.

The nurse developed a "salutogenic relationship" with Barbara. Beyond the traditional therapeutic relationship and its one-way flow of emotional intention and energy, the two-way flow of energy in the nurse's relationship with Barbara created a salutogenic phenomenon. The nurse's experience of coherence (commitment to her patient), manageability (persistence and success in her interactions), and meaning (mutual respect, trust, and affection) transformed her burnout. The New Year's Eve encounter with Barbara was a "salutogenic moment," in which the coherence created by her love of nursing and the intimate and profound interactions she experienced with Barbara led to a very different reaction to the trauma of that night. Salutogenic moments and relationships are not something "to do," but something to embrace, to let in. "I have faced challenges before, and they drive me deeper into my own self." In salutogenic experiences, a deep sense of coherence and meaning create a sense of manageability. This can have a profound protective effect in preventing burnout and treating it, especially with difficult or traumatic experiences or within a profession filled with chronic high levels of emotional labor. These moments are "vitamins for the soul" that enable nurses to continually develop a deep well of emotional resilience that encourages them to thrive.

APPLYING EI ABILITIES TO SALUTOGENESIS

EI abilities operationalize and facilitate salutogenic experiences and relationships. The four primary EI skills work together to do this, engaging emotional processes in the same way specific emotions have been illustrated in this text.

Using EI: Identifying Emotions/Emotional Phenomena

Experiencing coherence and meaning begins with paying attention to oneself, to one's own emotions and responses and being adept at one's own emotional phenomenology. In the crucible of her relationship with Barbara, the nurse realized that there was something beyond the frustration and struggle of the relationship. She embraced it as holy gift, a great teacher to her soul, and an unexpected help in a moment of professional crisis. Identifying emotions and emotional phenomena is a core skill for salutogenic practice. It is an invitation to the study of ones' own self. Paying attention is a first step in experiencing and going deeper into one's own coherence, meaning, and self-management.

Using EI: Understanding Emotions/Emotional Phenomena

By New Year's Day, the young nurse deeply understood the power of a fully engaged, therapeutic relationship. Her understanding of conflict, power struggles, and the energy of patients' fight for life, deepened across the months caring for this person. Her understanding moved beyond the apparent into the numinous, partially due to her acceptance of the gift of this difficult relationship. She would later say that Barbara was the exact medicine she needed to experience a deeper relationship with a patient than she had thought possible. It changed her permanently.

Using EI: Using Emotions/Emotional Phenomena to Reason and Managing Emotions/Emotional Phenomena

The nurse in this story integrated reasoning and emotions within the crucible of a difficult relationship. She accepted it as a gift, letting it work her and teach her. From the moment Barbara returned to the nurse's life, she realized this patient was a gift to her. She could fight it, she could even refuse the gift, but she could not deny the reality of it. There was nothing more sophisticated or elaborate than simply saying, "yes," letting it in, letting it work her, difficult and challenging as that felt. Her self-management in this difficult emotional situation was simply the decision to say "yes."

APPLYING EI TO SALUTOGENESIS IN COLLEGIAL RELATIONSHIPS

Collegial relationships, based on professional role interaction and shared values, commitment, and hardship can also be salutogenic. Two nurses who don't "get along" may find common ground (meaning) in shared commitment to solving a particularly difficult patient problem. A doctor and nurse may find new respect and a deeper level of effectiveness when they use their different approaches together to achieve a common goal, deepening their partnership at the same time patient goals are achieved. The effectiveness of excellent mentors, teachers, and supervisors often rest with their ability to form salutogenic relationships that are very different from friendships or other relationships of equal power.

In collegial relationships, EI ability feeds the salutogenic qualities of a relationship. Identifying emotions, especially those related to conflict like competitiveness, jealousy, defensiveness, and resistance leads to an opportunity to move beyond them and set shared meaning as the primary goal. This is illustrated in a relationship between two ICU nurses who openly acknowledged their dislike of each other. Head-to-head over a deep open wound in their patient's leg, they finally looked at each other and said, "You will never be my friend, but we both want this thing healed." This identification of emotions, along with the spoken commitment to a common goal, enabled them to set aside the emotions that were keeping them from working well together. They never did become friends, but their professional relationship, built on their mutual respect and professional work together, nourished them both.

EI, SALUTOGENESIS, AND NURSING RESEARCH

Little research examines EI ability as it affects salutogenesis in nurses specifically, but a great deal of evidence supports the relationship between EI and related concepts, physical and emotional health, self-efficacy, and emotional self-care in moral and spiritual distress. Meta-analysis of general population (including samples greater than 19,000), concluded that EI correlated with emotional and physical health (Kotsou et al., 2018; Martins et al., 2010). Development of EI ability has been correlated with health outcomes in nurses, and several studies identified EI as a mediator in nurses' stress responses and burnout (Afsar et al., 2017; Hurley et al., 2020; Jurado et al., 2019) (see Chapter 15 for research summary). It is particularly interesting that countries as culturally dissimilar as the United States, Pakistan, Greece, Spain, and China report similar findings.

DEVELOPING EMOTIONAL INTELLIGENCE AND CULTIVATING SALUTOGENESIS

SAMPLE EXERCISES #12A: THE PRACTICE OF REFLECTION AND USING THE RELAXATION RESPONSE

As the stories in this chapter suggest, identifying emotions in professional practice—and ways of understanding them, that have particularly rich meaning—is a great way to begin. Several questions can begin this practice. When you are at the bedside, what emotional experiences make you feel more human, more deeply alive? What emotions have the opposite effect, diminishing your humanity? What are the touchstone stories of your own life, the ones that ground the humanity of your professional practice? The ability to use emotions to reason is particularly important in this work. How does what I feel deepen my understanding of this emotion? How does my understanding of this emotion change how I feel?

SAMPLE EXERCISE 12B: USING THE RELAXATION RESPONSE

Many emotional wellness practices are based on physiological activation of the relaxation response (see Chapter 2). From intentional breathing, systematic muscular relaxation, meditation, and other mind-body awareness exercises, the relaxation response as a practice can be life-changing. Nurses can use EI abilities to support use of these practices. A simple example is noticing "I feel tense!" *Deep breath!* When a nurse identifies an emotion (tense, angry, anxious), understands that it has a body connection (tense neck, sore jaw), uses this emotion to reason ("Oh! My jaw is tense, that usually means I am angry.") and manage the emotion ("Okay, time for some stretching"), they can intentionally activate the relaxation response to decrease negative emotions and promote wellness.

Source: Benson, H. (2020). *Mind Body Institute*. https://www.bensonhenry institute.org/about-us-dr-herbert-benson/

REFERENCES

Afsar, B., Cheema, S., & Masood, M. (2017). The role of emotional dissonance and emotional intelligence on job-stress, burnout and well-being among nurses. *International Journal of Information Systems and Change Management, 9*(2), 87–105. https://doi.org/10.1504/IJISCM.2017.087952

Antonovsky, A. (1987). *Unraveling the mystery of health. How people manage stress and stay well*. Jossey-Bass.

Codier, E., Muneno, L., & Freitas, E. (2013). Emotional intelligence rounds: Developing emotional intelligence ability in clinical oncology nurses. *Oncology Nurse Forum, 40*(1), 22–29. https://doi.org/10.1188/13.ONF.22-29

Hurley, J., Hutchinson, M., Kozlowski, D., Gadd, M., & VanHorst, S. (2020). Emotional intelligence as a mechanism to build resilience and non technical skills in undergraduate nurses undertaking clinical placement. *International Journal of Mental Health Nursing, 29*(1), 47–55. https://doi.org/10.1111/inm .12607

Jurado, M. M. M., Pérez-Fuentes, M. C., Ruiz, N. F. O., Márquez, M. M. S., & Linares, J. J. G. (2019). Self-efficacy and emotional intelligence as predictors of perceived stress in nursing professionals. *Medicina (Lithuania), 55*(6). https:// doi.org/10.3390/medicina55060237

Kotsou, I., Mikolajczak, M., Heeren, A., Grégoire, J., & Leys, D. (2018). Improving emotional intelligence: A systematic review of existing work and future challenges. Emotion Review, 11(2), 151–165. https://doi.org/10.1177/ 1754073917735902

Martins, A., Ramalho, N., & Morin, E. (2010). A comprehensive meta-analysis of the relationship between emotional intelligence and health. *Personality and Individual Differences, 49*(6), 554–564. https://doi.org/10.1016/j.paid.2010.05 .029

Mayer, J. D., Caruso, D. R., & Salovey, P. (1999). Emotional intelligence meets traditional standards for an intelligence. *Intelligence, 27,* 267–298. https://doi .org/10.1016/S0160-2896(99)00016-1

Nurse.org. (2020). *News: Study reveals alarming statistics on nurse burnout: Report of National Nursing Engagement Report.* https://nurse.org/articles/nurse -burnout-statistics/

Santoft, F., Salomonsson, S., Hesser, H., Lindsater, E., Ljotsson, B., Lekander, G., Kecklund, G., Ost, L.-G., & Hedman-Lagerlöf, E. (2019). Mediators of change in cognitive behavior therapy for clinical burnout. *Behavior Therapy, 50*(3), 475–488. https://doi.org/10.1016/j.beth.2018.08.005

World Health Organization. (2019, May 28). *Burn-out an "occupational phenomenon": International Classification of Diseases.* https://www.who.int/mental _health/evidence/burn-out/en/#:~:text=Mental%20health%20publications -,Burn%2Dout%20an%20%22occupational%20phenomenon%22%3A %20International%20Classification%20of,classified%20as%20a%20medical %20condition

13

Emotional Intelligence
and Patient Safety

INTRODUCTION

Emotional intelligence (EI) is defined as the "ability to recognize the meanings of emotions ... and to reason and problem-solve on the basis of them" (Mayer et al., 1999, p. 267). In this chapter, EI is operationalized with the following skills:

1. Accurate identification of emotions in self and others
*2. Understanding emotions
*3. Using emotions to reason (integrating thinking and feeling)
4. Managing emotions
(Mayer et al., 1999).

*For the purposes of this chapter, skills 2 and 3 are reversed from the published order in Mayer et al. This better aligns the four abilities with the error management problem-solving processes discussed later in the chapter. Emotional intelligence (EI) offers a novel approach for addressing the ongoing patient safety crisis in the United States. In this chapter, several theoretical frameworks are utilized to illustrate EI abilities as a mechanism for the improvement of patient safety culture, the identification of clinical risk, and the reporting of error/near-miss events.

In addition to the ability EI Model, the following models and report mechanisms will be used to discuss EI's role in patient quality and safety:

1. The Healthcare Quality and Disparities Report (QDR)
2. The Reason Model of safety phenomena in clinical systems
3. Berlo's Communication Theory Model
4. The Emotional Intelligence in Patient Safety (EIPS) Model

PATIENT REPORTING OF QUALITY/SAFETY MEASURES IN THE UNITED STATES

In 1999, the U.S. Institute of Medicine (IOM) report on medical error, *To Err Is Human: Building a Safer Health System,* was a stunning wake-up call for healthcare professionals. The report estimated 100,000 patient deaths per annum as a result of medical error, a figure many later considered an underestimation (Kohn et al., 2000). Its publication signaled a sea change in U.S. healthcare delivery. Legislation was enacted to formalize accountability for and improvement in patient care quality and safety. One law stipulated the U.S. Congress receive an annual report on medical quality and safety indicators. The report, the National Healthcare QDR, is meant to provide an overview of the quality and safety of U.S. healthcare using specific quality and safety indicators. The report focuses on six major areas of health-care delivery, five of which address the safe delivery of care (Agency for Healthcare Research and Quality [AHRQ], 2018).

Across the United States, after the IOM report and subsequent legislation, patient care procedures, processes, and care culture were changed. Some improvement in safety metrics resulted. In 2019, the AHRQ reported that hospital-acquired conditions (HAC) resulting from care received between 2010 and 2016 had declined sharply, representing 3.1 million fewer incidences from the previous reporting period. It is estimated this prevented 125,000 deaths and saved an estimated 28 billion dollars (AHQR, 2016).

Despite such encouraging reports, there is, as of yet, no confidence that medical error statistics accurately reflect the full magnitude of the problem. A 2016 Johns Hopkins study estimated deaths from medical error at 250,000 per year, making medical error the third-leading cause of death in the United States. That study noted that death certificates do not include medical error as a cause of death, which contributes significantly to underreporting (Makary, 2016). Other research, published by the *Journal of Patient Safety*, estimated the annual error related to death figures as high as 440,000 (James, 2013).

The problem is not only patient deaths and inpatient care. Ten years after publication of the IOM study, it was estimated that out of every 1,000 U.S. hospital admissions, medical errors occurred in 115, at an estimated additional cost of $8,000 per admission (Shreve et al., 2010; Van Den Bos et al., 2011). In the outpatient setting, one study reported diagnostic test errors for 1 of every 20 outpatients, about half of which were identified as potentially harmful (James, 2013).

The emotional sequelae of medical errors are also serious and their consequences can be severe. In a Massachusetts medical error study, patients who had suffered a medical error within the previous 3 to 6 years were interviewed. Unsurprisingly, the study reported that 30% had avoided the responsible practitioner and institution. Moreover, these patients also reported having avoided healthcare, all healthcare, provided by anyone and anywhere, since the error event. The possible negative consequences this avoidance can create cannot be overstated. Negative emotional outcomes from medical errors often result when a patient is neither told about the error nor given a chance to discuss what happened and to have their questions answered (Betsy Lehman Center Commonwealth of Massachusetts, 2019). Many do not want compensation; they want closure.

Communication Error and EI

In the original IOM report, communication errors had been estimated to be causative or contributory factors in 80% of medical errors (Kohn et al., 2000). Although some improvements have been implemented, such as bedside shift change reports, specific communication education, performance goals, and objective performance criteria are generally lacking. A reference model for the role of communication and interpersonal relationships in patient safety is needed.

The 2018 QDR summary reflects data from hospital and outpatient care delivered between 2012 and 2016. Of the 36 patient safety measures examined, six require direct communication (such as patient teaching). In the 2018 QDR report, only one measure had improved since the previous study period. Of the remaining 30 indicators, nearly all can be negatively and indirectly affected by miscommunication, which is not tracked in any way by the QDR reporting system. These findings reflect the persistent role of communication error as a significant contributor to clinical safety errors (Kohn et al., 2000).

Communication, Emotional Intelligence, and Medical Procedure Errors

Conflict, miscommunication, and interpersonal problems among staff, patients, and families can result in medical errors. Even in something as basic as a medical procedure, simple emotional and communication errors can compromise patient safety. Every single medical procedure has three major phases: preparation, the procedure itself, and recovery. All medical procedures, from an intravenous catheter insertion to major surgery, have these phases in common. The factors related to safe procedural outcomes associated with each of the phases are also nearly universal. Figure 13.1 illustrates the relationship between these safety factors and communication error risk.

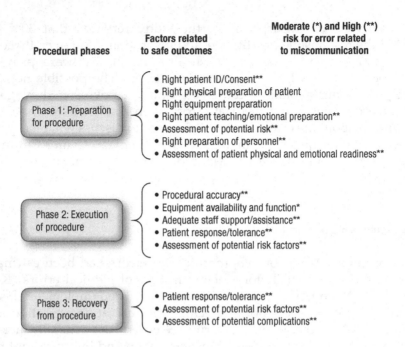

FIGURE 13.1 Procedural safety and miscommunication risk.

Story: Stuck Up

The patient in the medical/surgical unit was an elderly woman admitted for chronic obstructive pulmonary disease (COPD) with recent exacerbation. She had responded to initial care and had been relatively stable until she became mildly disoriented the day after admission. Her oxygen saturation levels were normal, but her heart rate and blood pressure were elevated. The staff, concerned about the possibility of hypercarbia and acid/base imbalance, notified the physician and received an order for an arterial blood gas (ABG) test.

The unit was busy. The patient's nurse was occupied with an acute admission. A respiratory therapist was called to perform the test. The therapist was a new hire and a recent graduate.

The patient was confused and uncooperative, and as a result, the therapist could not adequately immobilize the patient's arm for the procedure. The first and second blood draw attempts were unsuccessful. A senior therapist was called in for assistance for the third attempt, but because of a code in the emergency department, it took almost an hour before the senior therapist was available. By this time, the patient was acutely disoriented. The previous ABG draw attempts had left small hematomas, which had increased in size by the time the second therapist came from the ER. Only then did the therapist realize the patient was on anticoagulation therapy.

The nurse caring for the patient arrived just in time for the third ABG draw. She immediately expressed anger at the new therapist for "making a mess" of her patient, who was yelling and cursing the staff. The patient's disorientation made the third ABG attempt difficult, but the draw was successful. Unfortunately, the sample had to be thrown out when the results did not reflect the patient's true pulmonary status. Instead, they reflected respiratory alkalosis from the patient's screaming and hyperventilation. By the fourth ABG draw, the patient was unconscious. The last draw's findings revealed a severe combined respiratory and metabolic acidosis. Shortly after the results were called to the nursing unit, the patient coded.

Evaluation of Phase 1: Preparation for Procedure

Several safety factors listed in Figure 13.1 were compromised in Phase 1. It isn't clear if patient identification and consent were appropriate, but, given the baseline and progressive disorientation of the patient, both were likely inadequate. A patient who does not understand the necessity of the procedure they are about to undergo is already at risk, as their ability to cooperate with the procedure is compromised. In terms of the physical and emotional preparation of the patient, a patient with mental status changes may not be able to cooperate with or tolerate a painful procedure, increasing the safety risk. Further, the novice therapist did not prepare for this possibility by requesting assistance and sufficiently assessing the patient's physical and emotional readiness. Lastly, the assessment of physiological risk was poor. A COPD patient with exacerbation is at risk for both hypoxia and hypercarbia, and both can result in mental status deterioration. Additionally, nobody identified the patient was anticoagulated, placing the patient at risk for site hematoma under the best of conditions.

Even before the procedure, direct or indirect communication errors compromised numerous patient safety factors. Had the therapist communicated with the care team, a better assessment of the patient in preparation for the procedure could have taken place. Critical information regarding anticoagulants and the patient's ability to cooperate with the anticipated procedure could have been shared and a plan developed.

Evaluation of Phase 2: Execution of Procedure

The communication errors in Phase 1 carried over into Phase 2, the procedure itself. The result was two failed procedures, delayed treatment, and a complication. Due to the patient's anticoagulation status and likely inadequate compression of the two failed sites, hematomas formed. In the one-hour delay before the senior therapist arrived to do the (third) ABG draw attempt, the patient deteriorated. Her disorientation, hyperventilation, and yelling temporarily changed her condition by blowing off CO_2, so the successful (third) ABG draw did not reflect the patient's actual condition. By the fourth draw, the underlying physiological deterioration had overwhelmed the patient. The CO_2 level, having returned to the (prehyperventilation) high levels, resulted in a serious drop in the patient's level of consciousness and subsequent acute respiratory arrest.

Several risk factors for miscommunication were illustrated in this phase. Communication between the novice therapist, the nursing staff, and the senior respiratory therapist was clearly inadequate, resulting in delayed treatment and a serious negative outcome for the patient. When the nurse came to perform her own assessment, she wasted time and energy blaming the novice therapist. Effective teamwork with this newly unstable patient became even more challenging.

Evaluation of Phase 3: Procedure Recovery

Deterioration of the patient's condition resulted from a cascade of errors (see Figure 13.2). Like dominoes, the first communication error resulted in a series of subsequent errors. The result compromised not only procedural recovery but also the trajectory of the patient's acute illness.

Applying EI Abilities

Any experienced nurse would recognize the series of events in this story. It represents a common "Bermuda Triangle" of clinical phenomena: (1) a busy unit, (2) short staffing resulting from acuity changes on the unit and elsewhere in the hospital, and (3) team dysfunction, in this case exacerbated by a new, inexperienced team member. The cascade of

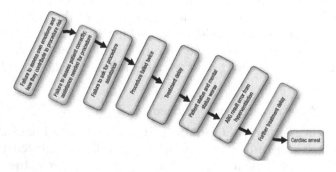

FIGURE 13.2 Procedure phase I: Error cascade.

miscommunication that can result in poor patient outcomes is not uncommon, begging the question, "Why do negative outcomes like this happen?" It is a given and understandable that novice practitioners are at higher risk for mismanaging critical clinical situations. Similarly, busy clinical units make communication more difficult. Unexpected admissions happen regularly, and when all staff are busy, it can be hard to get the needed assistance. But to accept this as the status quo is to accept negative outcomes as inevitable. Problems cannot be solved with the mindset that created them. Could thinking through this story using EI skills offer a different mindset?

Using EI: Identifying Emotions in Phase 1

What if the novice respiratory therapist had come into the situation explicitly aware of his own potential contribution to patient risk? New staff, especially professional novices, are often anxious to prove themselves as competent and independent. These emotions place them at high risk for not asking for help. The assumption that asking for help constitutes a kind of failure may have kept the novice therapist from being more insistent about asking for help or from going to the charge nurse or respiratory therapy supervisor for assistance.

An experienced, mature, and emotionally secure therapist, firmly grounded in a familiar interdisciplinary team, would not have hesitated to stick their head out of the patient's room to grab someone for help. "Hey, can I borrow you for a second?" could have made the procedure safer at the outset, and completely prevented the cascade of errors. But this novice therapist had a second major risk factor: they were new to the team. Without established relationships within their own department or interdisciplinary team, new staff cannot rely on developed interdisciplinary team skills. This places novice and new staff members at serious risk for inadequate communication. In this situation, a failure to communicate the need for assistance resulted at least in part because the therapist was unaware of their own emotional risk factors.

Using EI: Identifying Emotions to Reduce Risk, Phase 1

What if the therapist had checked their own emotions as a first step? What if, in the elevator on the way to the unit, they had taken a deep breath and said to themselves, *"Pulse check?* I am feeling anxious, eager to please, a bit nervous, and defensive. I want to prove myself." After realizing the situation required more than one person, a second pulse check would have been critical. "Oh, no! I am in a little over my head. I think I can do it, but is this safe? I want to prove myself, but maybe there is a nurses' aid who could help..." Even hitting the patient call button and asking for help would have mobilized the team. The clerk answering the call light would have then been responsible for finding someone on the team to help. An experienced team member would have both known to do this and felt comfortable doing so. That is what teams do for each other!

Using EI: Understanding Emotions in Phase I

What do we know about eagerness to prove competence, independence, and the ability to manage a difficult situation? These are natural emotions in both novice practitioners and those new to a team. Understanding the emotions means understanding that they are also high-risk emotions. If the therapist had consciously identified these emotions and applied their understanding of them, including the risks associated with them, they may have been able to choose a safer action. "OK! I am eager to prove myself, but that means I am trying too hard to be independent. This could be risky for the patient..."

What do we know about the desire to prove oneself to the team? "I don't need anyone; I never need help" does not generate confidence, respect, or good team function, while "Hey, I have a situation, can I borrow you for a minute?" is a better team builder. It communicates that a new person knows when they are overwhelmed, that they know when to ask for help, that they are willing to offer help to others, and that working together makes the team safer. The misconception that asking for help constitutes failure is one of the most insidious, pervasive, and common clinical culture elements that undermines patient safety.

Using EI: Using and Managing Emotions in Phase I

With a "pulse check" to identify emotions and with an understanding of them, the therapist could then use emotions to reason. Such emotional problem-solving could have changed the situation for the better. The novice therapist's emotional need to prove themselves overrode the need to ensure the safety of the patient. Put this way, it is a no-brainer. A split second of thought could have averted the cascade of error. The patient would have been safer, the novice could have had a positive clinical experience, and the team would have had a chance to grow stronger.

Getting help from the charge nurse, for example, could also have increased communication about other high-risk aspects. Catching key facts like the patient's anticoagulated status would have prevented another element of risk from escalating into additional patient injury. A third major event, the delay in treatment that resulted in a lab error, the need for a repeat procedure, and ultimately the patient's rapid physiological deterioration, could have been prevented. The "emotional pulse check" takes only seconds but can have a profound effect on a clinical outcome. In short, thinking differently about the clinical situation can create different outcomes. This simple illustration of using the four EI abilities in an early step in this situation illustrates how the use of EI could have prevented two of the negative safety events, the procedure failure and the resulting hematomas. (See Exhibit 13.1.)

EXHIBIT 13.1 Procedure Phase I: Use of EI To Improve Procedural Quality and Safety

Safety Indicators at Risk	EI Abilities to be Used	Changed Outcomes
-Right patient ID/Consent**	*Identify emotions in self and others	*Procedure failure averted
-Right physical patient preparation		*Hematomas averted
-Right equipment preparation	*Understand emotions	*Inaccurate lab results averted
-Right patient teaching/emotional care**	*Use emotions to reason	*One ABG stick instead of 4
-Assessment of potential risk**		*No treatment delay
-Right preparation of personnel**	*Manage emotions in self and in emotional situations	*Building of team
-Assessment of patient physical/emotional readiness**		*Positive experience for therapist

USING EI TO IMPROVE COMMUNICATION AND PATIENT SAFETY

Improving Patient Safety by Applying EI to Communication

A model for using EI to improve patient safety. In this model, EI skills mediate the relationship between communication and patient safety. In the model, Berlo's communication theory and Reason's model for safety performance are mediated by EI abilities. See Figure 13.3. This EIPS model (Emotional Intelligence in Patient Safety) suggests a means to improve patient safety.

Berlo posits both source and recipient of communication are influenced by communication knowledge, skills, attitudes, and the social/cultural context. When two people communicate or fail to, all these elements interact and affect communication effectiveness. All the elements can contribute to communication errors. Berlo also posits that emotions play a major part in this process. His theory identifies emotional capabilities and a wide range of positive and negative emotional factors that affect both the delivery and reception of communication content (Berlo, 1960).

Reason's model for safety performance within organizations, sometimes referred to as the "Swiss Cheese" model, describes the flow of

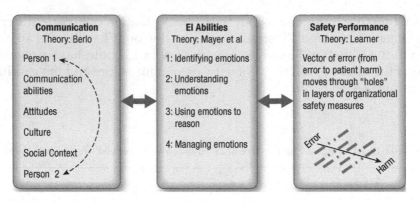

FIGURE 13.3 Procedure phase I: Use of EI to improve procedural quality and safety.
Source: Original to author

medical error events as an arrow moving from the error onset through to patient harm. This arrow moves through layers of safety mechanisms within an organization, through "holes" that result from safety breaches. When there are many or large "holes" in the system, risk for safety errors increase. This includes communication and interpersonal "holes" (Reason, 2000).

The EIPS model describes EI skills as a mediator between these two safety functions, communication and safety performance. (See Figure 13.3). In this model, EI skills influence the relationship between communication and safety in several ways. Effective communication itself is a safety system, as good communication within a team and among patients, families, and care providers make patients safer. In the Reason model, it creates a barrier to risk events, as shown in Figure 13.4 with a blue arrow, indicating a positive effect. Poor communication creates "holes" in this safety system. The direct negative effect is illustrated by a red arrow in Figure 13.4. Although there is little research on EI and patient safety, there is a lot of research (summarized in Chapter 15) of the relationship between EI ability and both communication and interpersonal effectiveness.

How EI Ability Improves Safety Indirectly

Strengthening safety systems: Improving communication strengthens safety systems within the clinical environment. For example, good staff relationships act as a safety system that can be made stronger and more resilient by EI skills. Staff are more apt to confront unsafe conditions if they have team support.

Hole gaps: EI abilities support identification and management of holes in safety systems. When a team with EI abilities find holes in the safety

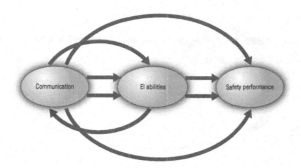

FIGURE 13.4 The EI/Patient Safety (EIPS) Model.
Sources: Berlo, D. (1960). *The process of communication.* Rinehart, & Winston; Mayer, J. D., Caruso, D., & Salovey, P. (1999). Emotional intelligence meets traditional standards for an intelligence. *Intelligence, 27,* 267–298. https://doi.org/10.1016/S0160-2896(99)00016-1; Reason, J. (2000). Human error: Models and management. *British Medical Journal, 320*(7237), 768–770. https://doi.org/10.1136/bmj.320.7237.768

system, their proper communication can decrease the probability these holes will result in a medical error. For example, if a unit has a hole in the form of a dysfunctional team member, the rest of the team can use EI abilities to effectively confront the poor practice to make the unit safer. When staff identify a high-risk process (a hole), effective EI skills help to more effectively change the organization.

Error management: When an error does occur, good communication, supported by EI abilities, decreases the emotional impact of the error, preventing long term patient harm. Effective communication about errors, particularly those from error-prone processes, helps strengthens safety mechanisms.

Improving safety culture: EI skills and communication skills mutually reinforce each other in a positive feedback loop of continuous improvement. As they strengthen and improve each other, risk (holes) are reduced and safety mechanisms within the organization are improved. These interactional effects are summarized in Figure 13.4.

APPLYING EI TO CHANGE THE CULTURE OF PATIENT SAFETY

Changing a culture prone to medical error is one of the most difficult obstacles to improving patient safety. In the traditional safety culture, blame and judgment undermine reporting and systems improvement. A "fix-the-problem-not-the-blame" approach is at least articulated if not operationalized in most healthcare organizations.

However, simply identifying risk management and quality improvement as a no-blame system is not enough to change a culture deeply ingrained in healthcare providers. The EIPS model may offer a way to

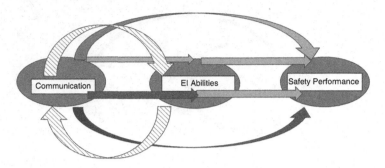

FIGURE 13.5 EI/Patient Safety (EIPS) Model.
In this model, good communication skills improve EI skills and good EI skills improve communication. These two skill sets are in a positive feedback loop. If communication skills are poor, EI abilities can improve them. If communication is poor, safety is compromised, but as EI ability improves communication, this negative influence is mitigated via EI abilities.

change the blame culture (see Figure 13.5). For example, in the story presented, several clinical culture issues predisposed the unit to the error. Using Reason's model, *the culture created holes* that made the flow from error to patient harm more likely, especially with the new employee orientation to the clinical unit.

Most clinical orientations are procedure/task-driven, give little or no attention to relationship building beyond superficial introductions, and tend to have "sink-or-swim" evaluations. How many orientations include a day where a respiratory therapist is paired with a nurse? What if integration into the team, either within a nursing team or an interdisciplinary team, was required in orientation? How much inter-shift conflict could be averted if new staff were required to orient to shifts to which they would not normally be assigned? Where intershift conflict exists, a "hole" has formed, and often a large one! Including EI skills for specific orientation objectives ("Identify three emotions that contribute to intershift conflict on your unit and discuss them with one member of each shift."), could also constitute a novel approach to improving clinical safety culture.

Another very common safety issue is the medical "lone ranger" culture. In a "lone ranger" culture, independence equals competence and asking for assistance indicates a failure. This is an endemic challenge to a culture of patient safety in the United States because of the value that individual skill and autonomy have over teamwork, collaboration, and standardization.

Although not illustrated in the story, a related issue is "macho" culture, when nurses routinely forego breaks, meals, and/or habitually stay late after their shift ends. Worse, not needing rest, food, bathroom breaks, or a scheduled departure are subtly not just tolerated but to some degree expected. A "macho" attitude equates these deprivations with high performance. All these common cultural features constitute cultural holes in safety systems. These systems depend on care, high levels of staff energy, focused attention, adaptability and responsiveness, and the ability to perceive subtle clinical changes, resist distraction and communicate effectively. Because of EI skills' ability to enhance all these qualities, basic EI skills can improve safety culture.

Story: Collecting Brains

Safety, quality care, and staff performance anxiety can be addressed with a culture of common values. One unit that worked frequently with clinical decisions based on complex hemodynamic variable assessments, adopted a phrase, "I need a second brain on this ... check me, OK?" This invited another nurse to look over a set of hemodynamic variables and validate their colleague's plan based on their own assessment. This simple phrase, "I need a second brain" encouraged a culture of collegial support of clinical decisions, helped novice staff to learn from more experienced staff, and prevented the implementation of poorly thought-out plans. For particularly high-risk situations, during a busy or short-staffed shift, or when a care provider wasn't thinking clearly, this phrase prevented errors and improved quality. To address the habit of skipping breaks and meals on a busy medical/surgical care unit, a nurse manager directed her intervention at the performance anxiety that usually drives this bad habit. When the staff did not take breaks or meals, it was referred to as a safety breach.

QSEN NURSE COMPETENCIES AND EMOTIONAL INTELLIGENCE NURSING RESEARCH

In 2003, the IOM published "Health Professions Education: A Bridge to Quality," which identified QSEN nurse competencies critical for safe, high-quality care. This document bridged patient safety and clinical practice by outlining specific nurse competencies that impact patient safety. These competencies focus on patient-centered care, teamwork and collaboration, evidence-based practice, quality improvement, safety, and informatics (Dolansky & Moore, 2013). These competencies depend on good communication and interpersonal skills and have a direct relationship with EI abilities. (See Table 13.1).

TABLE 13.1 QSEN Patient Safety Nurse Competencies and EI Abilities

QSEN COMPETENCY	EI ABILITIES	RESEARCH FOUNDATION
Patient-centered care	EI abilities correlate with patient-centered care outcomes	Strong
Teamwork	EI abilities relate to improved team outcomes, positive conflict resolution	Significant research across disciplines, little research in nursing
Collaboration	Because of the correlation with interpersonal skills and problem-solving, EI improves collaboration	Significant research across disciplines, little research in nursing
Evidence-based practice (EBP)	Because of the role of EI in change process, EI skills could support EBP	No research in nursing as of 2020
Quality improvement	Because of the role of EI in change process, risk assessment, and team skills, EI skills could support quality improvement	Little nursing research as of 2020
Safety	Because of the role of EI in change process, patient error follow-up, and reporting, EI skills could support improved safety	Little nursing research as of 2020; See EIPS Model
Informatics	Discussion of role of EI in informatics outside of nursing; little in nursing as of 2020	None

Source: Dolansky, M. A., & Moore, S. M. (2013). Quality and Safety Education for Nurses (QSEN): The key is systems thinking. *OJIN: The Online Journal of Issues in Nursing, 18*(3), 1.

DEVELOPING EMOTIONAL INTELLIGENCE TO IMPROVE PATIENT SAFETY AND QUALITY CARE

Sample Exercise #13: Using the EIPS Model, diagram a patient safety procedure on your unit that has an emotional or interpersonal "hole" in it. Describe how one EI ability could be used to ameliorate that hole.

REFERENCES

Agency for Healthcare Research and Quality. (2016, December). *National Scorecard on Rates of Hospital Acquired Conditions 2010 to 2015: Interim Data from National Efforts to Make HealthCare Safer.* https://www.ahrq.gov/hai/pfp/2015-interim .html

Agency for Healthcare Research and Quality. (2018, October). *National Healthcare Quality and Disparities Report: Chartbook on patient safety.* AHRQ Pub. No. 18(19)-0033-4-EF. https://www.ahrq.gov/sites/default/files/wysiwyg/research/ findings/nhqrdr/chartbooks/patientsafety/qdrpatientsafetychartbook-2017 update-090617.pdf

Berlo, D. (1960). *The process of communication.* Rinehart & Winston.

Betsy Lehman Center Commonwealth of Massachusetts. (2019). *The Financial and Human cost of medical error.* https://betsylehmancenterma.gov/assets/ uploads/Cost-of-Medical-Error-Report-2019.pdf

Codier, E., & Codier, D. (2015). A model for the role of emotional intelligence in patient safety. *Asia-Pacific Journal of Oncology Nursing, 2*(2), 112–117. https:// doi.org/10.4103/2347-5625.157594

Codier, E., & Codier, D. (2017). Could emotional intelligence make patients safer? *The American Journal of Nursing, 117*(7), 58–62. https://doi.org/10.1097/01.NAJ .0000520946.39224.db

Dolansky, M. A., & Moore, S. M. (2013). Quality and Safety Education for Nurses (QSEN): The key is systems thinking. *OJIN: The Online Journal of Issues in Nursing, 18*(3), Manuscript 1. https://doi.org/10.3912/OJIN.Vol18No03Man01

James, J. T. (2013). A new, evidence-based estimate of patient harms associated with hospital care. *Journal of Patient Safety, 9,* 122–128. https://doi.org/10.1097/ PTS.0b013e3182948a69

Kohn, L., Corrigan, J., & Donaldson, M. (2000). *To err is human: Building a safer health system.* Quality Chasm Series. National Academies Press. https:// www.nap.edu/catalog/9728/toerrishumanbuildingasaferhealthsystem

Makary, M. A. (2016). Medical error—The third leading cause of death in the US. *BMJ, 353,* i2139.

Mayer, J. D., Caruso, D., & Salovey, P. (1999). Emotional intelligence meets traditional standards for an intelligence. *Intelligence, 27,* 267–298. https://doi .org/10.1016/S0160-2896(99)00016-1

Reason, J. (2000). Human error: Models and management. *British Medical Journal, 320*(7237), 768–770. https://doi.org/10.1136/bmj.320.7237.768

Shreve, J., Van Den Bos, J., Gray, T., Halford, M., Rustagi, K., & Ziemkiewicz, E. (2010). *The economic measurement of medical errors.* Milliman, Inc. https://www .soa.org/Files/Research/Projects/research-econ-measurement.pdf

Van Den Bos, J., Rustagi, K., Gray, T., Halford, M., Ziemkiewicz, E., & Shreve, J. (2011). The $17.1 billion problem: The annual cost of measurable medical errors. *Health Affairs, 30*(4), 596–603. https://doi.org/10.1377/hlthaff.2011 .0084

14

Emotional Intelligence and Nursing Ethics

INTRODUCTION

In this chapter, emotional intelligence (EI) abilities are applied to ethics in nursing. EI abilities that operationally define the concepts are used as a framework:

1. Identifying emotions
2. Understanding emotions
3. Using emotions to reason
4. Managing emotions

The order of the EI abilities are modified from Mayer et al to better fit with nursing process (Mayer et al., 1999). These are applied to 3 aspects of nursing ethics:

1. Ethics in patient care
2. Ethics in care teams
3. Ethics in nurse self-care

A HISTORY OF NURSING ETHICS

The Nuremberg trials at the close of WWII offered disturbing questions. How can "good" people in traditionally honor-bound professions become complicit in some of the worst violations of humanity in history? What happens when individual professionals are not held to account by their peers, professions, and society as a whole? The trials showed how moral individuals within organizations can engage in morally "wrong" functions. "I was just following orders," complicit healthcare providers, doctors, and nurses claimed.

Morality refers to principles that help determine what is "right" and what is "wrong." Ethics is the related field that puts these principles to work to:

1. apply moral principles to choose "right" actions,
2. conduct relationships in an ethical manner, and
3. manage situations where a "right" action is clear but for some reason not possible.

The following principles are often applicable in healthcare:

Autonomy: This refers to a person's right to self-determination and independence. A patient is exercising autonomy when they choose treatments and goals for their care.

Fidelity: This relates to promises, commitments, truthfulness, and advocacy. Fidelity is applied when the care team does not withhold information from a patient. The relationship between nurse and patient, which is based on commitment and advocacy, is another example.

Nonmaleficence: "Do no harm," in the Hippocratic Oath and the Nightingale Pledge, as in choice of treatment with the lowest possibility of causing harm to a patient, like a drug with the fewest side effects, or not choosing a research treatment where risks outweigh benefits.

Beneficence: "Doing good," as in positive actions on another's behalf, like a nurse making a decision for their team that will result in the most benefits for the most people on the team.

Justice: Relating to fairness, this applies on both an individual and societal level. It posits that all people have, for example, rights to equal access to healthcare resources.

Paternalism: This principle involves taking over another's autonomy. A parent, for example, makes medical decisions for children; a spouse might for a cognitively impaired loved one. This principle has a challenging history in healthcare, as physicians guided by this principle historically "ordered" treatments and prescribed "what I think is best" for patients.

Utility: This principle applies to maximum usefulness and benefit, usually of resources of time, energy, material goods, and money. One aspect of utility is agent neutrality, which means that everyone is assumed to be equal in distribution of resources.

Source: Adapted from Iseminger et al. (2019).

Ethical Conflicts

Ethical conflicts occur when a moral principle is seriously violated or when two principles are in conflict. In one study, 60% of nurses surveyed reported that violations of autonomy and confidentiality were encountered daily in their practice (Ulrich et al., 2010). Conflict between principles can occur when two people are being motivated by two different beliefs. A physician acts on an idea of the "right" treatment for a patient and gets frustrated with a patient who has a different priority for their care. In this case, paternalism conflicts with autonomy. A nurse manager pleads for an increased budget for more staff to prevent burnout from mandatory overtime, but administration replies with "we don't have the resources." In this case, beneficence is trumped by utility.

Sometimes the conflict between principles occurs within one person! An ICU nurse may want to give her critically ill patient more time, even though she is caring for another patient. In this case, her desire to do "good" for her patient conflicts with the time, energy, and resources available. Here, beneficence conflicts with utility.

When ethical principles among a group collide, the ensuing conflict can be difficult to navigate even when all individuals have a clear or agreed upon goal. In settings such as oncology or critical care, where high-stakes treatment decisions are often ambiguous and end-of-life and treatment choices have ethical implications, this is common. Should the nearly dead suicide victim receive the last unit of O negative blood in the trauma unit, on Friday of a busy holiday weekend? Ethical conflicts can also occur when situational constraints render the "right" action impossible. A person expresses the desire to die at home, not in an ICU, but resources to support this are not available. The moral distress created by such dilemmas majorly contribute to nurse stress and burnout. The positive impact when such conflicts are resolved positively cannot be overstated.

Story: We Did It Right (For Once)

We had fought for his life for weeks, full court press, no holds barred, but he was dying. From the beginning, we all knew, as he did, his prognosis was not good. However, despite the severity of his condition, he had remained alert and cognitively intact. From the start he had said, "I am going to fight like hell, but if I have to die, I want to die at home."

When it became clear that we could not stop his death, we began preparations.

By this time, he was on a respirator, and continuous infusion drugs to maintain his blood pressure. He wrote on his communication pad, "If

I am going to die, I want to die in my own bed." He looked directly into our eyes as we read those words.

This was not possible. At the family conference, we proposed an alternative: taking him off the respirator, taking out the IV lines infusing his medications, and letting him be alone with his family for as long as possible to talk and be together. Everyone was on the same page, except at the conference's end, the family said, "We appreciate everything you all have done. We are so grateful. We just wish he could die at home as he requests." We each went back to our duties, our hearts heavy and sad.

No one remembers who first said it, but someone said two words that grew within the team like a seed: "Why not?" Ours was one of the best ICU teams around, with seasoned, experienced clinicians who had a history of advocating for our patients. If we could orchestrate a "good" death for him in our ICU, could we try the same for the death our patient wanted? What if, for once, our patient's choices overrode our need for control, rules, and protocols? One by one, team members asked, "Why not?" and proposed ideas for how they could help. It would be difficult, uncomfortable, and risky, but the team was unanimous. We all knew the downsides. He could die in the car in the parking lot. He could die in the few short miles to his house. We could not be there to help. Hospice and home care would not take responsibility for a 45-minute admission to their programs. The family and their friends would be on their own. Yet, at the next family conference, the family responded with tears of gratitude and relief. Our patient was clear, "At least I would die going home, even if I didn't make it to my bed."

It was the strangest ICU discharge. With all his life support machines and drugs, we rolled his ICU bed to the parking lot vehicle. He was tenderly lifted into the back seat of his family car, and we removed his respirator, IV lines, and all vestiges of his hospitalization. The driver hit the accelerator and they tore out of the parking lot. As we all watched this courageous family disappear from our lives, there was not a shred of sorrow among us. We were elated.

Hours later, the family called. He had peacefully died after hours laying in his bed, fading out of consciousness but with his family and friends around him.

We never did anything like that again, but the powerful joy of that experience stayed with each of us for years.

NURSING CODES OF ETHICS

Part of the Nuremberg trial's legacy was the subsequent development of professional codes of ethics across many professions, including nursing.

Until adoption of the first formal American Nurses Association (ANA) Code of Ethics in 1950, the only published ethical guide for nurses was the Nightingale Pledge, the nursing equivalent of the Hippocratic Oath. The pledge was not written by Florence Nightingale, who died in 1910. It was inspired by her and written by a committee coordinated by nurse Lystra Gretter in 1893, who revised it with an added phrase in 1935 to reflect the emerging role of nurses in public health (Gretter, 1893, in Fowler, 1984). The pledge reflects mostly "virtue" ethics or ethics of personal behavior and character, such as purity and devotion. Reference to moral principles is implied (see Box 14.1). Important as the pledge was to those who spoke their words at nursing school pledging ceremonies and graduations, the pledge carried no legal weight nor real consequences when violated.

BOX 14.1 The Nightingale Pledge, 1893 & 1935

VIRTUE TERMS IN THE PLEDGE	NIGHTINGALE PLEDGE (1893 AND 1935 VERSIONS)	MORAL PRINCIPLES IMPLIED
Purity	"I solemnly pledge myself before God and in the presence of this assembly, to pass my life in purity and to practice my profession faithfully. I will abstain from whatever is deleterious and mischievous and will not take or knowingly administer any harmful drug. I will do all in my power to maintain and elevate the standard of my profession, and will hold in confidence all personal matters committed to my keeping, and all family affairs coming to my knowledge in the practice of my calling. With loyalty will I endeavour to aid the physician in his work and devote myself to the welfare of those committed to my care." (Gretter, 1893, in Fowler, 1984)	
Faithfulness		Fidelity
Avoidance of mischievousness and anything deleterious		Non-malfeasance
Not take or administer any harmful drug		Non-malfeasance
Elevate standards of the profession		Fidelity
Confidentiality		Fidelity
Loyalty		Fidelity
Devotion to patients		Beneficence, Fidelity
	Added in 1935 … "and as a 'missioner of health' I will dedicate myself to devoted service to human welfare." (Gretter, 1935, in Fowler, 1984)	
Service to human welfare		Beneficence, Fidelity

Note: The spelling of endeavor is correct to the country and time of writing.
Source: Fowler, M. D. M. (1984). *Ethics and nursing, 1893-1984: The ideal of service, the reality of history* [Ph.D. thesis]. University of Southern California

In 1950, the first formalized ANA Code of Ethics established ethical practice as fundamental to nursing practice by placing it within the ANA document that defined what nursing is, how practice is defined, and its legal, social, and professional requirements. The code, and ethical competencies later derived from it, is considered "non-negotiable in all roles and in all settings" for every practicing nurse. Since its inception, the code has been adapted with new requirements and interpretive statements for nurse relationships, communication, human rights, and nurses' responsibility to care for themselves. The code is revised regularly as both the world and healthcare evolve.

From its roots in "virtue ethics," nursing ethics has evolved to a set of ethical practice competencies that require nurses to:

1. implement ethics in decision making,
2. understand ethical consequences of clinical decisions, and
3. integrate ethical issues in healthcare delivery, particularly to marginalized, vulnerable, and underserved populations.

EI Applied to the ANA Code of Ethics

The ANA Nursing Code of Ethics is all about ethics in relationships; relationships between nurses and patients, nurses and each other, nurses and other disciplines, nurses and organizations they work for, nurses and their communities, and last and most importantly, nurses and themselves. Emotional intelligence (EI) ability facilitates effectiveness in relationships, communication, conflict resolution, organizational and clinical outcomes, as well as personal self-efficacy. Because ethical challenges are so intrinsically emotional, EI abilities are important tools for developing ethics competencies and managing ethical conflicts.

There is general agreement that emotions play a significant role in ethical decision-making, but little research exists on how that actually works. Ethical competency appears to relate to emotional competency, as illustrated by the Ethical Competency Framework, inspired by early EI research. This competency framework reflects personal, social, and global ethical competencies, all of which are influenced by EI abilities. This model adapted for nursing practice is illustrated in Figure 14.1. This model makes it clear that for nurses, emotional competencies influence all aspects of ethical nursing practice, whether in a personal, social, professional, or global sphere of influence. For this reason, EI abilities provide nurses with a means to operationalize ethical competency in care of patients, work in teams, and as a means for self-care.

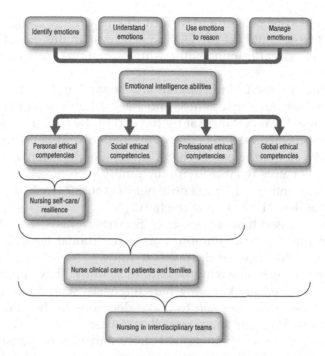

FIGURE 14.1 Ethical competency framework applied to EI in nursing practice.
Source: Adapted from Berghofer

EI APPLIED TO ETHICAL CARE OF PATIENTS

Story: Keeping Secrets

"As a novice nurse, and a newly independent young woman in my 20s, self-reliance was my personal and professional goal. When I first learned about ethics, I gravitated towards autonomy foremost. Patients should have the right to dictate their own destiny, fully participate in decisions about their care, and determine treatment goals. They needed to be fully and actively informed about their medical condition, and therefore, should always be told the truth. To me this was a no-brainer, as close to a universal ethical principle as I could imagine.

Not much later in my career, I was assigned to a very elderly Japanese woman, newly diagnosed with metastatic and likely fatal cancer. I was told in report she had not been included in discussions about her condition. Her family members, led by her son, represented her in the family meeting to discuss the findings of her work-up and likely choices for treatment. Although fully conscious and cognitively intact, she was kept in the dark about diagnosis and its likely trajectory.

I was livid. The patient had a right to know! How could the family not tell her? How could the physician participate in this ethical travesty? What was my ethical responsibility in this situation? How could I make this right?

I introduced myself to the patient and began her daily care. She was shy and reserved, but fully oriented and she gradually warmed to conversation with me. I was certain that by the end of the shift, I would be able to orchestrate a conversation between my patient and her doctor, even if her family did not participate. When I asked the physician about this, he clearly stated, 'I already talked with the family.'

'Doesn't she have a right to know her diagnosis?' I asked.

He responded, 'That is up to the family.'

Aghast, I pressed him on the issue, 'She has rights!'

He told me, 'This is common among traditional Japanese families. The family will decide what she needs to know.'

I later spent some time with the patient's family. They appreciated my concern but assured me knowing her diagnosis 'would just upset her.' She totally relied upon her son to make decisions for her. He loved his mother. He would ensure she was well cared for.

I believed them. Her son visited daily and was obviously very attached. He asked detailed questions about her care and followed up carefully when I asked about pain control and home care. But when I proposed including her in these discussions, he smiled gently and told me that he wanted to save his mother from any distress. 'I don't want her to worry,' he said, ending our talk.

This violated everything I knew about ethical care. Surely, she had a right to know what was happening. She should be able to choose priorities for the end of her own life! Clearly, it was time to talk with the patient directly. During a break in her care, I sat down next to her and asked pointedly, 'What do you know about your diagnosis? Has the doctor talked with you about this?'

The patient hesitated. 'My son takes care of these things.'

I pressed on, 'Would you like to be a part of the decisions that are made about your care?'

She responded again, 'It is up to my son. He understands these things.'

I tried one more time. 'The decisions that will be made in the next few days will affect the rest of your life a great deal. Isn't it important that you know as much as you can?'

She looked me directly in the eyes, and said, full of meaning, 'My son takes care of these things.'

I was taken aback because the message she was giving me was crystal clear: *Don't say anything more. I don't want to know.* I backed off immediately, shaken."

Story Reflection: The Anatomy of an Ethical Conflict

This story reflects a slippery slope common in medical ethics, the presumption that caregivers know what is "right" for patients. This is a typical form of paternalism, the ethical principle that reflects one person taking responsibility for another person. In this story, the physicians and the patient's son were motivated by paternalism, in both cases under the strong influence of beneficence, the desire to do good, and non-malfeasance, the desire to avoid harm. For many traditional Japanese families, paternalism is an important virtue. The danger of paternalism, however, is that it negates autonomy, the patients' right to determine for themselves, and the right to full information to be able to make their own decisions.

The nurse's distress had two origins. Most obviously, she saw the physician's and son's paternalism as negating the patient's autonomy. Less obviously, the nurse was also displaying paternalism when she presumed to know what was "right" for this patient, creating an ethical conflict within herself. Because autonomy was so important to her, she could not imagine it might not be important to her patient.

The patient was discharged to home and the family's care. The discharge teaching summary stated, "A family conference took place and the family is fully informed about the patient's diagnosis and care needs." The nurse waved good-bye to her patient, a knot in her stomach.

Ethical conflicts occur when ethical principles collide. In this case, autonomy, beneficence, and paternalism all conflicted. For a healthcare provider, ethical conflicts often create a "three-headed problem" (see Figure 14.2). The first "head" is risk to the patient, the second is risk to the team, and the third is risk to the care provider. The risks for each are different, each are problematic in different ways, and the negative effects of each can be significant and related to the other two. For patients, an ethical conflict can result in negative clinical outcomes. They might receive care they would not have chosen or consequences they would not have risked. For care teams, ethical conflicts can create team conflict, mistrust, poor communication, and disrupted team performance. For providers, ethical conflicts can create cognitive dissonance, a kind of psychological disequilibrium that creates physical and psychological symptoms. The resulting "moral distress" is a factor in caregiver burnout. This connection between morally ethical conflicts, moral distress, and nurse burnout is significant. Research findings demonstrate that confident nurses navigating morally complex situations have less moral distress and burnout (Rushton, 2016).

The story illustrates all three risk categories. The patient was potentially at risk for not being informed of her condition, not participating in care decisions, and disrupting family relationships. The care team was at odds as different ethical principles motivated the nurse and the doctor. Communication between team members was risked and again risked

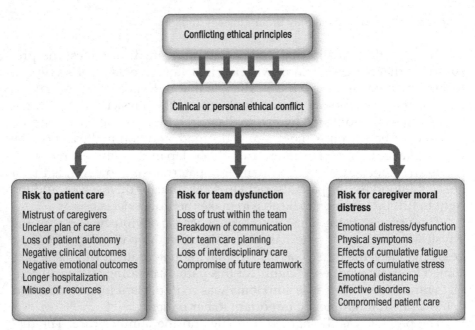

FIGURE 14.2 Anatomy of ethical conflicts.

when the nurse considered informing the patient of their condition. Undermining the physician was a real possibility. The nurse herself was at risk for moral distress when her motivating ethical principles, autonomy and truth telling, clashed with a family system that valued patient serenity over truth telling, and paternalism over autonomy.

EI Applied to Ethical Conflicts

Because of their positive effects on self-awareness, communication, and relationship management, EI abilities can be used to navigate ethical dilemmas, manage risk, and prevent negative effects to patient care, teams, and caregivers.

Using EI: Identifying Emotions

Identifying emotions is a great first step for managing ethical dilemmas. Questions like, "What am I feeling in the midst of this situation?" or, to another person, "What do you feel is most important?" can help identify the emotions engaged by the ethics of a situation. If the patient in the story had been asked, "What do you feel is most important for making health care decisions?" She likely would have reported being most comfortable and happy if she did not have to make them! A direct message like that would have clarified the situation. If the patient's son was asked the same question, he would likely have reported his mother's peace of mind was most important. If the nurse had asked the physician, "Do you feel any conflict between your responsibility to inform your patient and the cultural roles in this family?" they could have approached the situation more collaboratively. Lastly, if the nurse had inquired about her own feelings, the intensity of her distress, her emotional disconnect, and being at odds with everyone else in the situation, they could have been used as important information for emotional problem-solving.

Using EI: Understanding EI

Ethical conflicts are high-risk for charged emotional interactions because they are, by their nature, very personal. Passions can run high. Commonly, the focus turns to the caregiver's own ethical beliefs. Although they should not be dismissed, the ethical focus must primarily be on the patient. For this reason, emotional problem-solving in ethical dilemmas is important. After identifying the intensity and controversial nature of her own emotions, the nurse could have used this understanding as a "red flag" warning.

Understanding the emotional processes of traditional Japanese culture could also have supported in better understanding the family decisional dynamics. If the nurse had understood the son's fidelity and beneficence in its cultural context, she would have realized the patient's autonomy was not being usurped or controlled. For her patient, this was more important than her autonomy. It was autonomy as she understood it.

Using EI: Using EI to Reason

If the nurse identified her own emotions accurately, understood the risks of their intensity, and accepted that they were "out of step" with others in the situation, she could have used her emotions to reason through the situation differently. Ethical conflicts can feel personally threatening for care providers when personal values are challenged. However, while not insignificant, nurses' feelings in ethical conflicts cannot drive priorities of care. Remember, in healthcare ethical conflicts, the focus is the patient, not the care providers! If the nurse had used her emotions to reason, she would have realized that the patient supported the family's decision process. The patient had communicated she did not want to receive the information that the nurse was so anxious to give. The nurse's intense feelings grew out of her own ethical priorities, not the patient's. By using her emotions to reason, the nurse could have realized her own values actually threatened the ethical care of this patient.

Using EI: Managing Emotions

Identifying and understanding emotions and using them to reason could have helped this nurse manage herself and this emotional situation. If the conversation with the physician had begun, "It is so hard for me to see a patient kept in the dark like this," the physician may have shared his experiences with challenging cultural differences, maybe including strategies for dealing with it emotionally. With this sharing, the care team would have been stronger and more effective.

Her distress over the patient could have resolved into acceptance of this patient's values, although they were very different from her own. If the nurse had understood the conflict was within her own values, not her patient's, she could have gained a new cultural appreciation, confidence, and a deeper wisdom. This could have prepared her for similar situations in the future and decreased her risk for moral distress and burnout. The overall impact would have been not only a good clinical patient outcome, but a stronger team and a more mature, resilient nurse.

(NOTE: This story and reflection do not suggest nurse's ethical values should always be secondary to the patient's. If a nurse believes abortion is immoral, they should not participate in care of a patient who is having an abortion. It would be their professional responsibility not to work in a clinical setting where this would arise. Identifying this type of ethical constraint is professionally important, but such circumstances are less common than the types of conflicts described above.)

EI APPLIED TO ETHICAL PROBLEMS IN TEAMS

EI abilities can also support management of complex ethical issues in teams. This is particularly important for nurses who, research has shown, experience ethical dilemmas particularly acutely because of their central position in healthcare organizations, their diverse layers of responsibility, the systems of power, and loyalty ubiquitous to their roles (Chambliss, 1996).

Story: How Bad Can It Be?

A serious complication during a relative routine surgical procedure rendered a research unit's patient catastrophically brain damaged. The nursing staff caring for her had never cared for severe brain injuries. No one on the nursing staff had been involved with brain death workup and diagnosis. The legal determination of brain death was complicated by the local brain death statute, which was outdated and ambiguous. Disagreement between attending physicians delayed the patient's brain death diagnosis, and for several weeks the patient remained completely unresponsive but independently breathing.

During that time, the patient received the routine IV fluids and antibiotics ordered after surgery. Those treatments were not withdrawn, but no supportive treatments, such as nutrition and oxygen were ordered. The nursing staff was in shock and grieving the unexpected loss of their patient. Inexperienced in caring for neurologically damaged patients, they challenged the brain death diagnosis. Primitive reactions like startling to noise and following gaze, common in severe brain injury, were incorrectly interpreted as evidence of cognitive function. Disagreements and conflict developed about the patient's diagnosis and treatment plan. Emotions ran high, and the family received conflicting messages about their family member's condition.

The most religious nurses consulted with spiritual advisers and were told their religion demanded they support life and not participate in withdrawal of care for this patient. Some of these nurses began surreptitiously feeding the patient through her NG tube. Others wore prominent jewelry representative of their faith, a visible reflection of the "sides" of the conflict over this patient's care. The family, encouraged by the report from some nurses that "I know she can hear me," resisted any talk of cessation of supportive care or brain death determination.

Conflicts within the nursing team, the physician team, and the interdisciplinary team paralyzed the patient's care. Eventually, the patient was transferred to a hospital in a neighboring state with clear brain death criteria, where medical and nursing staffs were experienced in supporting family members throughout brain death diagnosis and withdrawal of life support. The brain death diagnosis was made quickly and the family was supported through treatment withdrawal.

Applying EI Abilities

EI abilities could have been useful in this situation in several ways. Risk factors for both team dysfunction and compromised patient care could have been identified and managed. Had this occurred, the ethical dilemma itself would have been easier to manage. Once the ethical conflict took root, EI abilities could have been used to manage the team conflict for better care for patient and family.

Using EI: Identification of Emotions
Even before the overt conflict over the ethical issues developed, identification of emotions could have supported the team. The unexpected

surgical complication severely shocked the entire interdisciplinary team, negatively affecting team performance. In this state, team members were unaware of the compromise of individual and team performance. Communication among team members and with the family was compromised. The family, without consistent messages from the interdisciplinary team, vacillated back and forth between "not wanting her to suffer anymore," and not wanting to "give up."

As the days passed and the shock began to wear off, the entire team grieved. This collective grief took many forms: anger, depression, anxiety, and even emotional withdrawal from other team members. This wide range of responses and the general unawareness of group grief on team functionality put the team emotionally out of step with each other. Most seriously, the staff did not identify the emotional risk that their grieving process had on family care and ethical decision-making. Their own unresolved emotions superseded clinical decision making, brain death determination, and the family's decision-making process.

Using EI: Understanding Emotions

The combined effects of shock, grief, and staff conflict resulted in emotional fatigue. Emotional thresholds for anger, anxiety, and frustration lowered. The team did not understand this was normal in light of the emotional trauma they were experiencing. Instead of "I am sorry I just snapped at you. My anger threshold is really low," the team engaged in blaming behavior and conflicts escalated regularly, sometimes over small clinical or unit management issues. Emotional conflict and polarized relationships undermined the diagnosis of brain death and rendered the family unsupported.

Using EI: Using EI to Reason and Managing Emotions

In this challenging and complex clinical situation, the emotions that impaired team function went unidentified. Understanding of the role of shock, grief, and conflict was not applied to the team's clinical functioning, and nobody engaged the "think/feel" process of using emotions to reason. Poor emotional problem-solving resulted and the situation was not managed effectively. Clinical care suffered and the patient's family was unnecessarily traumatized. Individual and team care failed.

EI AND THE ETHICS OF NURSING SELF-CARE

The early "virtue" ethics of nursing focused on duty, service, and implicitly, self-sacrifice. Inspired by these core virtues, nurses often find in their profession a way to live out values of service, care, and concern for others. But there is a "dark side" to the lineage: a denial of self-care. The ANA Ethics Code statement is remarkably clear: *Nurses have a duty to care for themselves as they do their patients.* Despite this, nurses chronically exhibit poor self-care (skipping breaks and meals) and accept hostile and unsupportive work environments (mandatory overtime). Most managers turn a blind eye to clear symptoms of burnout. As a breach in Ethics Code ethics itself, poor ethical climates also correlate with high-levels of moral distress, poor job satisfaction, and job turnover (Rushton, 2016).

This wound at the heart of nursing is rooted in nurses' concept of professionalism. This concept is formed around care of others without the *professional responsibility* to care for oneself, placing nurses at perpetual risk. The risk is not just to the nurse. A nurse who is neither resilient nor fully emotionally engaged risks patients as well. The "proper regard" for self-care, encoded in the ANA Code, requires nurses to accept emotional and ethical integrity as the foundation of their professionalism. Both necessitate integration of emotions into professional practice, something functionally discouraged in traditional healthcare systems.

Story: Hells Angel

As a critical care nurse educator orienting novice ICU nurses, I was doing rounds one day and found one of my students, a new grad orienting to the ICU, in the stairwell outside the unit, crying. Ann was one of my best students and had great promise to be an excellent ICU nurse. She was passionate, caring, inquisitive, an eager learner, and always up for a challenge. I asked her what was going on.

She said, "I can't be a nurse. I am unethical and unprofessional."

"What happened?" I asked.

Two Hells Angels motorcycle gang members had been riding together on one motorcycle when they collided with an 18-wheeler truck. One man was critically ill, very unstable, and the outlook for his survival was not good. His friend in the ICU room next door had minor injuries. Ann was caring for the second crash victim. He was hostile and uncooperative, refusing some meds and treatments. He even wore his "Hells Angels" jacket over his hospital issue gown. Distrustful and uncommunicative with doctors and nurses alike, he pretended not to notice the flurry of activity in his friend's room, but he got quiet when the activity abruptly stopped, and the team left his friend's room. His friend had died, and no one on the team knew how to tell him. Ann was taking his vital signs when he asked, "My friend just died, didn't he?"

In the stairwell, Ann said, "I never had to deal with something like this before. I didn't know what to say. His friend had just died. What could I say? It was so sad!" I asked her what happened next. She said, "I sat down on his bed. I was trying to figure out how to tell him, and I couldn't help it, a tear fell down my face. It was just so sad." She paused before saying, "I know this was unethical. I was so unprofessional. I will resign today. Don't worry."

I was stunned and heart-broken listening to this excellent nurse. Ann epitomized professionalism in everything she did. I quietly asked, "What happened next?"

She wiped her eyes. "He put his head on my shoulder and started to cry himself. He just sobbed."

"Do you know what therapeutic use of self is?" I asked. At Ann's blank look, I told her what I understood from her story. First, this man was someone no one else could reach, who trusted no one on staff, yet he trusted her to confirm his friend's death. Second, her tear of sadness in the face of horrible grief released her patient's grief. He was able to express his pain and get support, all because of the tear that ran down her cheek. Far from being unprofessional, or unethical, that tear was powerful medicine.

We talked about therapeutic use of self, the idea that who the nurse is and the fullness of their personality and experience and emotions can be medicine for patients. I explained to Ann that the story she told was an example of this powerful kind of nurse professionalism.

EI Abilities Applied to Ethics and Professionalism

There is a pervasive myth in nursing that nurses must be unemotional to be professional and that to express their emotions is not only unprofessional, but unethical and a violation of the "virtue ethics" of selflessness and caring for others. Implicitly, nurses with personal emotional issues should "leave it at home" as if they can place their feelings in their hospital locker on the way to work. For the shifts with emotional challenges, the unspoken rule is "don't take it home with you" as if the same locker gets filled with the day's unresolved feelings. This myth can create habits of emotional distancing and detachment even in instances where emotional connection and expressiveness could be life-giving to patients. Emotions cannot be set aside like a bagged lunch and soiled shoes, and this expectation places nurses at risk for moral distress, emotional dysfunction, burnout, and the poor patient care and team function that result.

If, on the other hand, emotions are accepted as part of self-care, team care, and patient care, professionalism takes on a more full, vibrant, and life-giving dimension. When nurses' emotional expressions are beneficent (working for the best good for the patient), when they are a function of fidelity (the nurse's promise of caring for the patient), and when it does no harm, they can be a strong force for healing and comfort for their patient. At the same time, effective identification of a nurse's own emotions, understanding them, using them to reason, and then managing them makes the nurse stronger, wiser, and more resilient.

Using EI: Identifying Emotions

Emotional expressions are not always beneficial or appropriate, so identifying emotions accurately is important. To identify that mounting frustration at a patient's lack of cooperation has now shifted to anger and impatience within the nurse, it would prevent an emotional expression that would wound the patient and disrupt the therapeutic relationship. That emotional expression would violate ethical principles of beneficence and nonmaleficence.

In the story however, feeling the sadness of the situation, and the appropriate expression of the sadness, resulted in a positive patient outcome. This was particularly important because of the patient's emotional detachment and mistrust, and his previous unwillingness to accept information, let alone comfort and support.

Using EI: Understanding Emotions and Using Them to Reason

Intuitively, this nurse understood grief as an emotion that forges emotional connection. Sitting with this hostile, uncooperative man and sharing her sadness enabled the therapeutic relationship to "work." This understanding also helped ensure emotional sharing was "beneficent" in the patient's best interest.

Using EI: Managing Emotions

It is a common assumption that "managing" emotions implies controlling them. However, this story illustrates the opposite, the power of simple emotional expression. Particularly in high-charged situations, authentic expression of emotions can be powerful in themselves as well as offering modeling for patients. Ann's behavior said, "grief is okay," and freed her patient to feel and express his own grief.

Applying EI to Nursing Care of the Nurse

The earliest references to ethical practice in nursing were nursing "virtues" such as honesty and caring. Although the nine statements in the

ANA Code of Ethics include "virtue ethics," they also include responsibility for understanding and applying complex ethical concepts as well as the remarkable statement that nurses have a duty to "care for themselves as they care for patients" (ANA, 2015). Despite this, nurses routinely skip meals, don't take breaks, risk physical injury moving patients without help, work mandatory double shifts, and tolerate work environments that are sometimes abusive and hostile. The culture of nursing, with its foundation of caring, service, and self-sacrifice often unwittingly supports this. Managers and hospital administrators, for whom these behaviors solve problems (understaffing, sick calls, unexpected admissions), often accept these "self-care violations" as routine and acceptable. To create a thriving professional life, nurses must not only be proactive with self-care, but also confront working habits, behaviors, and environments that subvert appropriate self-care. EI abilities can be used to both identify proactive self-care activities and confront working behaviors and conditions that undermine nurse thriving.

Using EI: Identifying Emotions

Noticing feelings is a self-care habit. Identifying emotions accurately builds self-care habits and helps in recognizing work habits and conditions that undermine nurse thriving. A nurse might notice a certain creative activity makes them feel happy, relaxed, and less stressed. Building the activity into a self-care habit starts with identifying emotions. At work, an uncharacteristic feeling of resentment might be a "red flag" for a nurse pressured to skip breaks and meals on a perpetually busy unit. Noticing resentment as information is the first step to break the habit of subverting self-care in a situation that will always reward that. Nurses should ask themselves, "What do you feel like when you are thriving?" Similarly, nurses should know the emotional symptoms of burnout, like negativity, emotional distancing, sarcasm, and avoidance and they should be able to identify it in themselves and others.

Using EI: Understanding Emotions

Understanding emotions protects self-care habits. For example, emotional thresholds rise when a person thrives emotionally. In emotionally challenging workplaces, maintaining emotional resilience keeps thresholds high. Chronic fatigue, stress, or crisis deplete emotional energy, lowering emotional thresholds. Nurses in these situations more quickly feel anger, frustration, and emotional distress. Nurses must also understand what creates and sustains burnout. Its risk factors, like social isolation, relationship breakdown, physiological changes, and chronic stress associated with it must be understood for nurses to be proactive at burnout prevention as well as early identification and treatment.

Using EI: Using EI to Reason and Management of Emotions

When emotions are identified accurately and understood, nurses can approach emotional problem-solving with "think/feel" skills. Thinking can inform feelings and feelings can inform thinking, particularly with burnout prevention and treatment. A trauma nurse identified early signs of burnout in herself. Friends and family said, "Go somewhere with a slower pace where you can take it easy for a while. Go do something you already know. You don't have the energy right now to learn something new."

While this advice made sense, she separately realized her burnout was mostly related to the "high tech death" she confronted daily. She had always believed in the dignity and integrity of the dying process, but ICU death violated that. By integrating her thinking and feeling, she realized her burnout began with losing her belief in a "good death." She transferred to a hospice unit with a specific goal of restoring her faith in a "good death." Self-care requires emotional management and planning to both promote thriving self-care plan and also management of work conditions that undermine nurse thriving.

RESEARCH ON ETHICS AND EI

Little research exists that explores the relationship between EI and ethics competencies. One study concluded that EI abilities were predictors of ethics competencies (Dangmei & Singh, 2017). In another, nurses confident in ethically challenging care had less moral distress and burnout (Rushton, 2016).

DEVELOPING NURSING EMOTIONAL INTELLIGENCE IN ETHICS CARE

SAMPLE EMOTIONAL DEVELOPMENT EXERCISE #14: USING EMOTIONAL INTELLIGENCE TO REACH ETHICS

Teaching ethics to nurses is challenging. The material itself, with its arcane language and definitions can provide an obstacle for student learning. Using EI abilities as a framework for analyzing an ethical dilemma can be one useful tool (Table 14.1).

TABLE 14.1 EI Development: Sample 14: Using Preprogrammed Avatars to Teach Ethics

AVATAR ROLE AND DIALOGUE	WHAT IS THIS PERSON FOCUSING ON EMOTIONALLY?	ASSOCIATED ETHICAL PRINCIPLE	IMPLICATIONS
Patient: "I have been a good wife and tried to be a good mother to you all. But this cancer has really taken it out of me and I am tired of fighting. I know you all have strong feelings about my decision to stop treatment but it is my choice."	This woman is standing up for herself. She is tired of fighting.	Autonomy	This patient always tried to be good to others (beneficence). Now she is claiming her right to decide on the basis of her needs, not others (autonomy).
Son: You have always been so good to us and we love you so much. I don't know what we will do without you to take care of us. But we have also been good Catholics, and to stop treatment is a way of you killing yourself. Self-harm is a sin!"	Concern about self-harm Concern about losing her care for them	Nonmaleficence Paternalism	It is important to this person that an authority outside the family have moral authority over decision-making. This constitutes a challenge to patient autonomy.
Husband: "I promised you that I would always take care of you no matter what. I would never want you to be in pain or suffering and even though I hate to let you go, I made you a promise to care for you according to your wishes."	Responsibility to his wife and his commitments to her	Fidelity	His highest priority is doing the right thing according to her wishes.
Doctor: "I have told you over and over again that the best thing for you to do is accept the treatment that I have suggested. I know what is best for cases like yours."	Sees the treatment choice as his to recommend	Paternalism	"The best thing" also reflects the desire to do what is right.
Nurse: "It doesn't seem right to pressure this woman into treatment when there are others who need the treatment resources. Others could benefit from treatment she doesn't want."	Thinking about distribution of resources and fairness	Justice	Interested in the best good for the most people.

REFERENCES

American Nurses Association. (2015). *Code of ethics for nurses with interpretive statements.* Nursesbooks.org. www.nursingworld.org/MainMenuCategories/EthicsStandards/CodeofEthicsforNurses/Code-of-Ethics-For-Nurses.html

Berghofer, D. (n.d.). *The ethical competence framework: Introduction.* The Institute for Ethical Leadership. http://ethicalleadership.com/content/Ethical%20Competence%20Framework%20Intro.pdf

Chambliss, D. F. (1956). *The social organization of ethics (morality and society series).* The University of Chicago Press.

Dangmei, J., & Singh, A. P. (2017). Relationship between emotional intelligence and ethical competence: An empirical study. *International Journal of Management, IT & Engineering, 7*(12), 119.

Fowler, M. D. M. (1984). *Ethics and nursing, 1893-1984: The ideal of service, the reality of history* [Ph.D. thesis]. University of Southern California.

Gretter, L. (1893). *The Florence Nightingale pledge.* https://www.truthaboutnursing.org/press/pioneers/nightingale_pledge.html#gsc.tab=0

Iseminger, K., Kemeryu, S., & White, L. M. (2019). Ethics. In J. K. Payne & K. Murphy-Ende (Eds.), *Current trends in oncology nursing* (2nd ed.). Oncology Nursing Society.

Mayer, J. D., Caruso, D., & Salovey, P. (1999). Emotional intelligence meets traditional standards for an intelligence. *Intelligence, 27,* 267–298. https://doi.org/10.1016/S0160-2896(99)00016-1

Rushton, C. M. (2016). Moral resilience: A capacity for navigating moral distress in critical care. *AACN Advanced Critical Care, 27*(1), 111–119. https://doi.org/10.4037/aacnacc2016275

Ulrich, C. M., Taylor, C., Soeken, K., O'Donnell, P., Farrar, A., Danis, M., & Grady, C. (2010). Everyday ethics: Ethical issues and stress in nursing practice. *Journal of Advanced Nursing, 66*(11), 2510–2519. https://doi.org/10.1111/j.1365-2648.2010.05425.x

15

Review of 20 Years of Nurse Emotional Intelligence Research, 1999–2019

INTRODUCTION

This chapter describes an overview of the first 20 years of nursing Emotional Intelligence (EI) research. The following questions are addressed: (1) How did the volume of nursing EI research studies change across the first 20 years? (2) How did the international nursing community contribute to this body of research? (3) How did type of research, methodology, and sample sizes change across this period? (4) What EI models and instrumentation were utilized? (5) What variables were explored? and (6) What observations does the descriptive review offer?

EMOTIONAL INTELLIGENCE IN THE NURSING LITERATURE: THE BEGINNING

The first nursing EI research study was published in 1999 (dos Santos et al., 1999). This new research field in nursing built on over a decade of EI research in other fields. Ten years after publication of the first nursing study, a review of the first decade of nursing EI research reported that, of the 39 nurse EI publications reviewed, 21 were editorial, four were opinion pieces, and nine were reports of empirical studies (Bulmer-Smith et al., 2009).

The earliest nursing EI research was descriptive and correlational, had simple designs and relatively small sample sizes. Much of it was exploratory in nature, examining EI's possible relevance to nursing. These studies generally validated findings from research in other disciplines, which had already published evidence of the correlation between EI and performance, teamwork, leadership effectiveness, customer satisfaction, stress management, burnout prevention, wellness parameters and positive fiscal outcomes. Preliminary nursing research demonstrated similar findings. Early nursing EI research also demonstrated correlation between EI and variables of particular importance to nursing: burnout prevention, perceived stress, organizational commitment, team function, emotional and physical wellness, customer satisfaction, fiscal outcomes, positive conflict styles, and greater resilience during organizational change. For nurse researchers, these findings were simply too compelling to ignore.

Early nursing EI research focused on a few basic questions:

- Is EI a part of nursing practice?
- Does EI correlate with important aspects of nursing, like clinical performance, retention, burnout, and leadership?
- If EI correlates with these things, is it therefore an important concept for nursing?

An example of research from this time was a descriptive analysis of 75 stories that nurses had written about nursing. The stories were evaluated by a team of researchers to see if the stories demonstrated EI attributes. Only one story did not, and of those that did, an average of four EI attributes were found per story. The number of attributes per story also correlated with degree of professionalism and level practice ranked by each of the researchers (Codier et al., 2010).

LITERATURE REVIEW OF NURSING EI RESEARCH, 1999–2019

As the body of nurse EI research developed, research study sample sizes, range of study variables, sophistication of methodology, and data analysis all increased. To describe this evolution in more detail, a combined Scopus search and snowball methodology was undertaken to describe 20 years of nursing EI research. Over 500 published studies were reviewed, inclusion criteria applied, and a descriptive analysis performed on the studies that met review criteria.

Purpose

The literature review focused on a 20-year period beginning with the first published EI nursing research study in 1999 and ending with the last study published in 2019. The goal was descriptive rather than meta-analytical, focusing on changes in volume of published research, international contributions, and evolution of research methodology such as the type of research, sample sizes, and variables explored. A general description of areas of strength and weakness in the body of evidence was undertaken.

Inclusion/Exclusion Criteria and Descriptive Variables:

1. A formal research question had to be posed as well as a specific methodology (qualitative, quantitative, or mixed).
2. The first author had to be a nurse.
3. EI had to be either a primary focus of the research or one of the primary variables studied.
4. The population of the study had to be nurses only; interprofessional population studies were excluded.
5. Quantitative research had to use a measure of EI; qualitative studies had to utilize a specific EI model.
6. Only published findings were included; dissertations were not included.
7. Relevant findings had to be reported.
8. The research had to be available to the reviewer.
9. If not published in English, English abstracts or article summaries had to be available.

The review constitutes only a reflection, not a comprehensive report of existing nurse EI research during this period.

Data Collection

Search terms included "Nursing" and "Emotional Intelligence." Snowball criteria included "Emotional Intelligence" and some aspect of nursing in the research article title. The initial search produced just over 500 articles. About half met inclusion criteria.

The following information was compiled for each:

- Date of publication
- Study purpose (variables examined in the study)
- Discipline of journal/book in which the research was published
- Nation in which the study took place
- Research method
- Sample and findings and the EI model used (including the EI instrument used, if used)

Studies were included even if not all this information was available.

Findings

Countries Publishing Nursing Research

By the end of December 2019, 40 countries had published at least one nursing EI research study. The fact that only English language articles or abstracts were included distorts the picture of the state of the nursing research. China, Jordan, and Spain, for example, all published significantly more research than was available in English. Spain and the United States were early leaders in nurse EI research, publishing 21 and 23 studies respectively across the twenty-year period. Starting in 2007, almost every year at least one nursing EI study was published in Spain and the United States. Over the twenty-year period, the following countries published greater than 10 studies: Turkey, South Korea, Iran, and Australia. Countries that published two to nine nurse EI studies included Canada, China, the United Kingdom, Japan, Ghana, and South Africa. By 2019, at least one nurse EI research study had been published by an additional 28 countries.

Volume of Nursing Research

From 1999–2019, the number of nursing EI studies published annually increased steadily. Fewer than three studies were published yearly from 1999 to 2007. From 2007 on, the total number of studies published annually increased almost every year. The annual number of EI nurse research studies reached double digits by 2013 and in 2019 exceeded 30.

Sample Size and Research Methods

In early nursing EI research, sample sizes were for the most part small, and most methodologies were correlational, descriptive, and exploratory. As research evidence correlating EI to nursing gradually grew, so did sample sizes and sophistication of study methodologies. Prior to 2014, studies reporting sample sizes of less than 100 participants outnumbered those with sample sizes greater than 100. This trend reversed beginning in 2014 and has held for every year following. In 2019, more than half the published studies had sample sizes of over 200. Three studies, in 2014, 2015, and 2018, reported sample sizes of over a thousand.

Study methodology also evolved. From 2009 onward, more published research utilized complex variable relationships, multivariate analysis, and even predictive modeling. After 10 years of research, studies of the body of evidence itself had begun. By the end of 2019 over a dozen surveys of nursing EI research, literature, integrative reviews, and meta-analysis had been published.

Models and Instrumentation

A variety of EI models and instruments are represented in the nursing literature reviewed. Instruments ranged from those requiring researcher certification (MSCEIT, v2, for example) to instruments created by study researchers. The validity and reliability of instruments ranged from rigorous to untested. Some studies discussed conceptual distinctions (ability model versus trait model versus mixed model) while others did not. Instruments that required certification for administration or those only available for purchase created limitations on their use. This was likely a substantive factor in the selection of study instrumentation. This constitutes a serious limitation in the research, as financial restrictions for nurse researchers most likely resulted in use of inferior instruments, like self-report instruments, for example. Similarly, EI models may have been chosen simply because a corresponding instrument was easily available.

Variables Investigated

The most frequent topics of interest were, in descending order:

1. Student EI
2. Nurse stress, burnout, resilience and other self-care variables
3. EI and nurse leadership
4. Interpersonal variables (communication, caring, conflict).

Only a few studies focused on nurse performance, retention, patient clinical outcomes, nursing instructor EI, or patient safety.

Nursing EI Literature Reviews, Integrative Reviews, and Meta-analysis

By the time the body of nursing research had developed to the point where analysis and description of the existing literature was appropriate, numerous meta-analysis on a variety of subjects already existed in the general literature of other disciplines (Martins et al., 2010; Van Rooy & Viswesvaran, 2004). By 2019, nearly a dozen meta-analysis, literature reviews, concept analysis, and integrative reviews had been published on EI and some aspect of nursing. One of the earliest reviewed a small body of early nursing EI research literature (Bulmer-Smith et al., 2009). Later reviews were topic-specific, providing evidence for the importance of EI as a concept for clinical and student nursing, nurse leadership, emotional caring of patients, moderating nurse work stress, better overall nurse health, increased work satisfaction, decreased risk of job burnout, and less moral distress in end-of-life care (Lewis, 2019; Nightengale et al., 2018; Prezerakos, 2018; Raghubir, 2018).

A 2019 meta-analysis of 12 nursing studies evaluating the importance of EI for nursing concluded that (1) EI ability is important for clinical practice (based on its correlation with performance, retention, commitment, career longevity, work wellness, and career longevity), (2) EI ability in nurses is important organizationally (because of its relationship with team and interdisciplinary practice), and (3) A variety of EI programs or techniques improved measured EI in nurses (Faria et al., 2019).

EVIDENCE FOR EI IN NURSING

The strongest evidence for the importance of EI in nursing practice falls into the following five findings categories:

1. Relationship between EI and clinical or organizational performance
2. Relationship of EI with nurse wellness, burnout, and emotional health
3. Patient outcomes and safety
4. Nursing education
5. Methods for developing EI abilities

In this section, for clarity of presentation, only the most recent research references are included. Supporting studies from earlier in the 20-year period are included under topical headings in the Suggested Reading section.

EI as Related to Clinical and Organizational Performance

Job performance and organizational variables were among the earliest EI research published in disciplines outside nursing. The resulting body of evidence formed a solid base for nursing EI research, which has provided evidence for a relationship between EI and nurse clinical performance (Al-Hamdan et al., 2017; Geun & Park, 2019; Harper & Schnek, 2012; Heydari et al., 2016).

There is also evidence that nurse EI correlates with caring, effective communication, engagement with patients, and interpersonal skills. This includes physical, emotional, and cognitive effectiveness; nurse ownership of and engagement with care; and critical thinking and emotional problem-solving (Ghasemi et al., 2018; Giménez-Espert & Prado-Gascó, 2018; Perez-Fuentes et al., 2018; Yanis et al., 2019). Additional references from earlier in the 20-year period are listed topically in the reference section.

There is evidence for the relationship between EI and organizational performance indicators, including job satisfaction, professional behavior, psychological empowerment, job retention, patient satisfaction, work engagement, organizational commitment, job conscientiousness, civic virtue, altruism, courtesy, and organizational citizenship behaviors (Celik, 2017; Geun & Park, 2019; Kim & Lee, 2019; Mohamed et al., 2017). See reference list for earlier supporting references.

Interdisciplinary research indicates a positive effect of EI on team performance, which has been validated in nursing (Jordan & Troth, 2002; Quoidbach & Hanseene, 2009).

Building on a significant body of evidence from other disciplines, however, the relationship between EI ability and nurse leadership effectiveness is substantial and of sufficient volume to have been explored in several meta-analysis (Akerjordet & Severinsson, 2008, 2018; Vitello-Cicciuo, 2002). The performance and organizational nurse EI research is particularly striking, as similar research findings have been reported across disparate cultures from countries as different as the United States, Jordan, China, Iran, South Korea, and Greece.

EI AND NURSE WELLNESS, STRESS, AND BURNOUT

In 2010, a multidisciplinary meta-analysis on employee EI and wellness included 19,815 participants and reported a positive relationship between EI and health (Martins et al., 2010). Nurse EI research has reported similar findings (Karimi et al., 2014), including one study in which EI was statistically predictive of nurse work wellness (Nel et al., 2014).

Numerous nursing studies have reported an inverse relationship between EI and both perceived stress and burnout in nurses (Afsar et al., 2018; Szczygiel & Mikolajczak, 2018). The mediating effect of EI on other variable relationships has also been demonstrated, such as between perfectionism and burnout, work effort and fatigue, and between strong negative emotions and burnout. The predictive role of EI for burnout and well-being has been demonstrated (de Loof et al., 2019). Work/life balance correlated at low, medium, and high levels with EI (Susi et al., 2019).

EI AND CLINICAL PATIENT OUTCOMES, SAFETY, AND PATIENT SATISFACTION

Relatively few nurse EI studies have explored specific patient outcomes, but the findings of those few suggest the importance of further study. Early nurse EI research demonstrated evidence for the relationship between EI and patient satisfaction and hospital services quality (Oyur, 2017). Although models for the relationship between EI ability and patient safety have been explicated, no nursing research has so far explored this. A few studies have reported correlation between nurse EI with clinical outcomes such as rates of infection, patient falls, glycemic control in diabetics, and medication compliance in HIV infected patients (Adams & Isler, 2014; Akbarilakeh et al., 2018; Jeffs et al., 2018; Mirzaei et al., 2019).

General wellness and quality of life has been correlated with EI in diabetic and hemodialysis patients (Samar, 2001; Shahnavazi et al., 2012). Measured EI of breast cancer survivors was a predictor of both physical and mental health (Mirzaei et al., 2019). Qualitative evidence suggests the importance of EI in nurse executives' success in leading quality and safety initiatives (Jeffs et al., 2018). Similar findings have been reported from countries as different as the United States, Iran, Turkey, and Canada.

EMOTIONAL INTELLIGENCE IN NURSING EDUCATION

Nursing students are ready and available research subjects. In the Nursing EI research from 1999 to 2019, research on student nurses significantly outnumbered any other nursing EI research topic. Numerous nursing studies have provided evidence for the positive impact of EI on academic success and completion of a nursing program, measured by academic, clinical, and standardized testing measures (Banjar & Seesy, 2019; Kim & Sohn, 2019; Rode & Brown, 2019). In one study, EI correlated significantly with three critical elements of nursing student success: academic achievement, clinical achievement, and retention in the nursing school program (Kim & Sohn, 2019).

Evidence also supports a direct correlation between EI and student nurse leadership, problem-focused coping, critical thinking, caring behavior, subjective well-being, mental health, interpersonal relationships, communication, avoidance of high-risk health behaviors, academic procrastination, and satisfaction with clinical experiences. An inverse relationship with perceived stress was repeatedly demonstrated (Akbarilakeh et al., 2018; Madadkhani & Nikoogoftar, 2015; Sharon & Grinberg, 2018; Yanis et al., 2019).

DEVELOPING THE EI OF NURSES

Numerous studies in the general literature suggest EI can be improved with a wide range of training methods. A review of the general literature in 2018 analyzed 46 studies across many disciplines and supported this conclusion (Yanis et al., 2019). A developing body of nurse EI research supports the same conclusion for both nursing student and practicing nurse populations. Interventions among the nursing studies included peer coaching, EI training sessions, problem-solving training, group support, didactic EI classes, EI training videos, peer counseling, peer coaching, journaling, and reflection. These findings have been demonstrated across numerous cultures and across clinical settings as diverse as caring post-operative patients, geriatric populations, and cancer care (Kikanloo et al., 2019; Kotsou et al., 2018; Kozolowski et al., 2018; Shenghong et al., 2019).

There is conflicting data on the effect of nursing schools on student EI (Cheshire et al., 2015; Di Lorenzo et al., 2019; Foster et al., 2017; Sharon & Grinberg, 2018). Very little research exists on nursing instructor EI.

SUMMARY OF THE 1999–2019 DESCRIPTIVE ANALYSIS

The body of nursing EI research grew and developed steadily over its first 20 years. The size, sophistication, and range of topics evolved steadily over this period. The number of countries involved in nurse EI research is impressive, and several countries produced EI nurse research leaders. The nursing EI research in this period included (1) multiple research studies on important topics, such as the correlation between EI and nursing performance, (2) studies that confirmed findings in the EI general literature, and (3) a dozen literature reviews and meta-analysis. The question, "Is emotional intelligence an important concept for nursing?" appears, on the basis of the first 20 years of research, to be answered with a resounding, "Yes!" Of particular significance are studies from countries across the globe, representing disparate cultures but focusing on similar research questions, reported similar findings. It is particularly significant when similar studies from the United States, Jordan, China, the United Kingdom, and Iran come to similar conclusions about a topic that has such varied cultural implications across cultures. Is EI a common phenomenon in nursing across cultures?

In nursing EI research overall and in other disciplines, significant theoretical disagreement abounds over the definition of EI. Varied EI models continue to be used that differ conceptually and operationally.

As in the general EI research, use of varying EI concepts, operational definitions, and instrumentation methods continues to be a challenge. The instruments used to measure EI vary widely from self-report to 360-degree feedback, and to ability testing. The validity and reliability of these instruments vary, creating an "apples and oranges" problem when trying to compare research studies. If two studies on performance, for example, come to the same conclusions but were based on very different conceptual definitions of EI and very different ways of measuring it, were the findings of these two studies legitimately inter-validating? It would seem not.

Economic and resource access problems are also likely and probably present an ongoing challenge for nurse EI research. The most rigorously tested EI instruments require researcher certification and are only available for purchase. Nurse researchers without the resources to obtain them must use instruments with less established validity and reliability.

One of the troubling observations of this review of the literature was an anecdotal observation. Not many EI researchers published more than one EI study, raising difficult questions: Is EI research difficult to fund? As an innovative topic and new concept, are faculty in the academic setting discouraged from pursuing it as a primary field of research? Is mentoring and guidance unavailable for those interested in studying this new field in nursing? Is the research undermined by the necessity of using instruments with poorly documented validity and reliability?

Opportunities ahead for EI research include the following: (1) Topics: Nursing research on nurse performance, retention, safety, patient outcomes should be developed; (2) Conceptual development: The challenge ahead for nursing is to develop a coherent and consistent, well-tested, validated model for EI in nursing, along with accessible instrumentation that can be used to measure it. Until this is accomplished, the "apples and oranges" problem in the body of nurse EI research will continue; and (3) Funding and administrative support: High quality research in nursing must be supported with time, energy, resources, and mentoring. This is challenging with new concepts and cutting-edge ideas, particularly those that challenge existing ideas, methods, and policies. A new generation of courageous leaders have an opportunity to challenge existing nursing school admission methods, for example, and both PhD programs and faculty developers have the chance to encourage faculty to focus their careers on EI.

REFERENCES

Adams, K., & Iseler, J. I. (2014). The relationship of bedside nurses' emotional intelligence with quality of care. *Journal of Nursing Care Quality, 29*(2), 174–181. https://doi.org/10.1097/NCQ.0000000000000039

Afsar, B., Cheema, S., & Masood, M. (2018). The role of emotional dissonance and emotional intelligence on job-stress, burnout and well-being among nurses. *International Journal of Information Systems and Change Management, 9*(2), 187–105. https://doi.org/10.1504/IJISCM.2017.087952

Akbarilakeh, M., Naderi, A., & Arbabisarjou, A. (2018). Critical thinking and emotional intelligence skills and relationship with students' academic achievement. *Prensa Medica Argentina, 104*(2), 1000280. https://doi.org/10.4172/lpma.1000280

Akerjordet, K., & Severinsson, E. (2008). Emotionally intelligent nurse leadership: A literature review study. *Journal of Nursing Management, 16*(5), 565–577. https://doi.org/10.1111/J.1365-2834.2008.00893.x

Akerjordet, K., & Severinsson, E. (2018). The state of the science of emotional intelligence related to nursing leadership: An integrative review. *Journal of Nursing Management, 18*(4), 363–382. https://doi.org/10.1111/J.1365-2834.2010.01087.x

Al-Hamdan, Z., Oweidat, I., Al-Faouri, I., & Codier, E. (2017). Correlating emotional intelligence and job performance among Jordanian hospitals' registered nurses. *Nursing Forum, 52*(1), 12–20. https://doi.org/10.1111/nuf.12160

Banjar, H., & Seesy, N. (2019). Measurement of the emotional intelligence competencies for effective leaders among Saudi nursing students at King Abdul Al Aziz University. *American Journal of Nursing Research, 7*(4), 420–427. https://doi.org/10.12691/ajnr-7-4-3

Bulmer Smith, K., Profetto McGrath, J., & Cummings, G. (2009). Emotional intelligence and nursing: An integrative literature review. *International*

Journal of Nursing Studies, 46, 1624–1636. https://doi.org/10.1016/j.ijnurstu
.2009.05.024

Çelik, G. O. (2017). The relationship between patient satisfaction and emotional
intelligence skills of nurses working in surgical clinics. *Patient Preference and
Adherence, 11,* 1363–1368. https://doi.org/10.2147/PPA.S136185

Cheshire, M. H., Strickland, H. P., & Carter, M. R. (2015). Comparing traditional
measures of academic success with emotional intelligence scores in nursing
students. *Asia-Pacific Journal of Oncology Nursing, 2*(2), 99–106. https://doi.org/
10.4103/2347-5625.154090

Codier, E., Muneno, L., Franey, K., & Matsuura, F. (2010). Is emotional intelligence
an important concept for nurses? *Journal of Psychiatric and Mental Health
Nursing, 17*(10), 940–948. https://doi.org/10.1111/j.1365-2850.2010.01610.x

de Looff, P., Didden, R., Embregts, P., & Nijman, H. (2019). Burnout symptoms in
forensic mental health nurses: Results from a longitudinal study. *International
Journal of Mental Health Nursing, 28*(1), 306–317. https://doi.org/10.1111/inm.12536

Di Lorenzo, R., Venturelli, G., Spiga, G., & Ferri, P. (2019). Emotional intelligence,
empathy and alexithymia: A cross-sectional survey on emotional competence
in a group of nursing students, *Acta Biomed for Health Professions, 90*(4), 32–43.
https://doi.org/10.23750/abm.v90i4-S.8273

dos Santos, L. M., de Almeida, F. L., & da Costa Lemos, S. (1999). Emotional
intelligence: Testing the future nursing. *Revista Brasileira de Enfermagem,
52*(3), 401–412. https://doi.org/10.1590/s0034-71671999000300010

Faria, N., Ramalhal, T., & Bernardes Lucas, P. (2019). Scoping review: The
emotional intelligence of nurses in the clinical care environment. *Annals of
Medicine, 5*(Suppl. 1), 206. https://doi.org/10.1080/07853890.2018.1560166

Foster, K., Fethney, J., McKenzie, H., Fisher, M., Harkness, E., & Kozlowski, D.
(2017). Emotional intelligence increases over time: A longitudinal study of
Australian pre-registration nursing students. *Nurse Education Today, 55,* 65–
70. https://doi.org/10.1016/j.nedt.2017.05.008

Geun, H., & Park, E. (2019). Influence of emotional intelligence, communication,
and organizational commitment on nursing productivity among Korean
nurses. *Journal of Korean Academy of Community Health Nursing, 30*(2), 226–
233. https://doi.org/10.12799/jkachn.2019.30.2.226

Ghasemi, S. S., Olyaie, N., & Shami, S. (2018). An investigation into the correlation
between emotional intelligence and communication skills among nursing
students. *Indian Journal of Forensic Medicine and Toxicology, 12*(3), 178–183.
https://doi.org/10.5958/0973-9130.2018.00155.X

Giménez-Espert, M. D. C., & Prado-Gascó, V. J. (2018). The role of empathy and
emotional intelligence in nurses' communication attitudes using regression
models and fuzzy-set qualitative comparative analysis models. *Journal of
Clinical Nursing, 27*(13–14), 2661–2672. https://doi.org/10.1111/jocn.14325

Harper, M. G., & Schenk, J. (2012). The emotional intelligence profile of successful
staff nurses. *Journal of Continuing Education in Nursing, 43*(8), 354–362. https://
doi.org/10.3928/00220124-20120615-44

Heydari, A., Kareshiki, H., & Armat, M. (2016). Is nurses' professional competence
related to their personality and emotional intelligence? A cross-sectional
study. *Journal of Caring Sciences, 5*(2), 121–132. https://doi.org/10.15171/jcs
.2016.013

Jeffs, L., Baker, G., Taggar, R., Hubley, P. B., Richards, J., Merkley, J., Shearer, J., Webster, H., Dizon, M., & Fong, J. H. (2018). Attributes and actions required to advance quality and safety in hospitals: Insights from nurse executives. *Nursing Leadership, 31*(2), 20–31. https://doi.org/10.12927/cjnl.2018.25606

Jordan, P. J., & Troth, A. C. (2002). Emotional intelligence and conflict resolution in nursing. *Contemporary Nurse, 13*(1), 94–100. https://doi.org/10.5172/conu.13.1.94

Karimi, L., Leggat, S. G., Donohue, L., Farrell, G., & Couper, G. E. (2014). Emotional rescue: The role of emotional intelligence and emotional labour on well-being and job-stress among community nurses. *Journal of Advanced Nursing, 70*(1), 176–186. https://doi.org/10.1111/jan.12185

Kikanloo, A. A., Jalali, K., Asadi, K., Shokrpour, N., Amiri, M., & Bazrafkan, L. (2019). Emotional intelligence skills: Is nurses' stress and professional competence related to their emotional intelligence training? A quasi experimental study. *Journal of Advances in Medical Education and Professionalism, 7*(3), 138–143. https://doi.org/10.30476/jamp.2019.74922

Kim, S., & Sohn, S. K. (2019). Emotional intelligence, problem solving ability, self-efficacy, and clinical performance among nursing students: A structural equation model. *Korean Journal of Adult Nursing, 31*(4), 380–388. https://doi.org/10.7475/kjan.2019.31.4.380

Kotsou, I., Mikolajczak, M., Heeren, A., Grégoire, J., & Leys, D. (2018). Improving emotional intelligence: A systematic review of existing work and future challenges. *Emotion Review, 11*(2), 151–165. https://doi.org/10.1177/1754073917735902

Kozolowski, D., Hutchernson, M., & Hurley, J. (2018). Increasing nurses' emotional intelligence with a brief intervention. *Journal of Quality Care, 29*(2), 59–61. https://doi.org/10.1016/j.apnr.2018.04.001

Lewis, S. (2019). Emotional intelligence in neonatal intensive care unit nurses: Decreasing moral distress in end-of-life care and laying a foundation for improved outcomes: An integrative review. *Journal of Hospice and Palliative Nursing, 21*(4), 250–256. https://doi.org/10.1097/njh.0000000000000561

Madadkhani, Z., & Nikoogoftar, M. (2015). Critical thinking in nurses: Predictive role of emotional intelligence. *Hayat, 4*(8), 77–88.

Martins, A., Ramalho, N., & Morin, E. (2010). A comprehensive meta-analysis of the relationship between emotional intelligence and health. *Personality and Individual Differences, 49*(6), 554–564. https://doi.org/10.1016/j.paid.2010.05.029

Mirzaei, S., Tame, A. I., Anabiaie, E., Moradipour, F., Nasiri, M., & Rohani, C. (2019). Emotional intelligence as a predictor of health-related quality of life in breast cancer survivors. *Asia Pacific Journal of Oncology Nursing, 6*(3), 261–268. https://doi.org.10.4103/apjpn.apjon_76_18

Mohamed, H. A., Mahmoud, S. M., & Mohamed, S. A. (2017). Psychological empowerment, emotional intelligence and professional behavior among nurse interns. *IOSR Journal of Nursing and Health Science, 6*(2), 112–121. https://doi.org/10.9790/1959-060202112121

Nel, J. A., Jonker, C. S., & Rabie, T. (2014). Emotional intelligence and wellness among employees working in the nursing environment. *Journal of Psychology in Africa, 23*(2), 195–203. https://doi.org/10.1080/14330237.2013.10820615

Nightengale, S., Spiby, H., Sheen, K., & Slade, P. (2018). The impact of emotional intelligence in health care professionals on caring behavior towards patients in clinical and long-term care settings: Findings from an integrative review. *International Journal of Nursing Studies, 80*, 106–117. https://doi.org/10.1016/j.ijnurstu.2018.01.006

Oyur, C. G. (2017). The relationship between patient satisfaction and emotional intelligence skills of nurses working in surgical clinics. *Patient Preference and Adherence, 11*, 1363–1368. https://doi.org/10.2147/PPA.S136185

Perez-Fuentes, M., del Mar Molero Juardo, M., Linares, J., & Reves, N. (2018). The role of emotional intelligence in engagement in nurses. *International Journal of Environmental Research and Public Health, 15*(9), 1915. https://doi.org/10.3390/ijerph15091915

Prezerakos, P. E. (2018). Nurse managers' emotional intelligence and effective leadership: A review of the current evidence. *Open Nursing Journal, 12*(1), 86–92. https://doi.org/10.2174/1874434601812010086

Quoidbach, J., & Hansenne, M. (2009). The impact of trait emotional intelligence on nursing team performance and cohesiveness. *Journal of Professional Nursing, 25*(1), 23–29. https://doi.org/10.1016/j.profnurs.2007.12.002

Raghubir, A. E. (2018). Emotional intelligence in professional nursing practice: A concept review using Rodgers's evolutionary analysis approach. *International Journal of Nursing Sciences, 5*(2), 126–130. https://doi.org/10.1016/j.ijnss.2018.03.004

Rode, J., & Brown, K. (2019). Emotional intelligence relates to NCLEX and standardized readiness test. *Nurse Educator, 44*(3), 154–158. https://doi.org/10.1097/nne.0000000000000565

Samar, A. D. (2001). *The relationship among emotional intelligence, self-management and glycemic control in individuals with type 1 diabetes* [Doctoral dissertations, University of Massachusetts Amherst]. Proquest. Paper AAI3012180.

Shahnavazi, M., Parsa-Yekta, Z., Yekaninejad, M., Amaniyan, S., Griffiths, P., & Vaismoradi, M. (2018). The effect of the emotional intelligence education programme on quality of life in haemodialysis patients. *Applied Nursing Research, 39*, 18–25. https://doi.org/10.1016/j.apnr.2017.10.017

Sharon, D., & Grinberg, K. (2018). Does the level of emotional intelligence affect the degree of success in nursing studies? *Nurse Education Today, 64*, 21–26. https://doi.org/10.1016/j.nedt.2018.01.030

Susi, S., Jothikumar, R., & Suresh, A. (2019). Collision of emotional intelligence and work centrality on work-life balance—A supportive work environment for working professionals. *International Journal of Environment and Waste Management, 24*(3), 250–258. https://doi.org/10.1504/IJEWM.2019.103102

Szczygiel, D., & Mikolajczak, M. (2018). Emotional intelligence buffers the effects of negative emotions on job burnout in nursing. *Frontiers in Psychology, 9*, 2649. https://doi.org/10.3389/fpsyg.2018.02649

Van Rooy, D. L., & Viswesvaran, C. (2004). Emotional intelligence: A meta-analytic investigation of predicative validity and nomological net. *Journal Vocation Behaviour, 65*, 71–95. https://doi.org/10.1016/S0001-8791(03)00076-9

Vitello-Cicciuo, J. M. (2002). Exploring emotional intelligence: Implications for nursing leaders. *Journal of Nursing Administration, 32*(4), 203–210. https://doi.org/10.1097/00005110-200204000-00009

Yanis, K., Lavia, P., & Nursalam, L. (2019). Factors affecting Nurse Caring Behaviors in Surabaya Jemursari Islamic Hospitals Indian. *Journal of Public Health research and Development, 10*(8), 3621–3636. https://doi.org/10.5958/0976-55062019.022655.4

SUGGESTED ADDITIONAL READING

EI and Literature Reviews

Lewis, G. M., Neville, C., & Ashkanasy, N. M. (2017). Emotional intelligence and affective events in nurse education: A narrative review. *Nurse Education Today, 53*, 34–40. https://doi.org/10.1016/j.nedt.2017.04.001

Powell, K. R., Mabry, J., & Mixer, S. (2015). Emotional intelligence: A critical evaluation of the literature with implications for mental health nursing leadership. *Issues in Mental Health Nursing, 36*(5), 346–356. https://doi.org/10.3109/01612840.2014.994079

Symeou, M., Efstathiou, A., & Jelastopulu, E. (2016). Exploring the relationship between emotional intelligence and job-stress in nursing personnel. *Hellenic Journal of Nursing, 55*(2), 149–157.

Thomas, D. S., & Natarajan, J. R. (2017). Emotional intelligence among nursing students—An integrated review. *Journal of Nursing and Health Science, 6*(1), 81–89. https://doi.org/10.9790/19590601078189

EI and Performance, Retention, Job Satisfaction

Bakr, M., & Safaan, S. (2012). Emotional intelligence: A key for nurses' performance. *Journal of American Science, 8*(11), 385–393.

Cho, H., Choi, Y., Jeon, M., & Jung, G. (2015). Factors affecting nursing productivity of clinical nurses: Focused on emotional intelligence and burnout. *The Journal of the Korea Contents Association, 15*(9), 307–316. https://doi.org/10.5392/JKCA.2015.15.09.307

Codier, E., Kamika, C., Kooker, B. M., & Shoultz, J. (2009). Emotional intelligence: Performance and retention. *Nursing Administration Quarterly, 33*(4), 310–316. https://doi.org/10.1097/NAQ.0b013e3181b9dd5d

Codier, E., Kooker, B. M., & Shoultz, J. (2008). Measuring the emotional intelligence of clinical staff nurses an approach for improving the clinical care environment. *Nursing Administration Quarterly, 32*(1), 8–14. https://doi.org/10.1097/01.NAQ.0000305942.38816.3b

Fujino, Y., Tanaka, M., Yonemitsu, Y., & Kawamoto, R. (2014). The relationship between characteristics of nursing performance and years of experience in nurses with high emotional intelligence. *International Journal of Nursing Practice, 21*(6), 876–881. https://doi.org/10.1111/ijn.12311

Mrayyan, M., & Al-Faouri, I. (2008). Predictors of career commitment and job performance of Jordanian nurses. *Journal of Nursing Management, 16*(3), 246–256. https://doi.org/10.1111/J.1744-6198.2008.00092.x

Tagoe, T., & Quarshie, E. N.-B. (2017). The relationship between emotional intelligence and job satisfaction among nurses in Accra. *Nursing Open, 4*(2), 84–89. https://doi.org/10.1002/nop2.70

Thomas, D. S., & Natarajan, J. R. (2017). Emotional intelligence among nursing students—An integrated review. *Journal of Nursing and Health Science, 6*(1), 81–89. https://doi.org/10.9790/1959-0601078189

Toyama, H., & Mauno, S.(2016). A latent profile analysis of trait emotional intelligence to identify beneficial and risk profiles in well-being and job performance: A study among Japanese eldercare nurses. *International Journal of Work Organization and Emotion, 7*(4), 336–353. https://doi.org/10.1504/IJWOE.2016.081841

Trivellasa, P., Gerogiannisb, V., & Svarnab, S. (2013). Exploring workplace implications of emotional intelligence (WLEIS) in hospitals: Job satisfaction and turnover intention. *Procedia - Social and Behavioral Sciences, 73*, 701–709. https://doi.org/10.1016/j.sbspro.2013.02.108

EI and Caring, Communication, Interpersonal Relationships

Hajibabaee, F., Farahani, A. M., Ameri, Z., Salehi, T., & Hosseini, F. (2018). The relationship between empathy and emotional intelligence among Iranian nursing students. *International Journal of Medical Education, 9*, 239–243. https://doi.org/10.5116/ijme.5b83.e2a5

Hutchinson, M., Hurley, J., Kozlowski, D., & Whitehair, L. (2017). The use of emotional intelligence capabilities in clinical reasoning and decision-making: A qualitative, exploratory study. *Journal of Clinical Nursing, 27*(3–4), e600–e610. https://doi.org/10.1111/jocn.14106

Kaur, D. M., & Kumar, N. (2015). The impact of emotional intelligence and spiritual intelligence on the caring behavior of nurses: A dimension-level exploratory study among public hospitals in Malaysia. *Applied Nursing Research, 28*(4), 293–298. https://doi.org/10.1016/j.apnr.2015.01.006

Ko, H. R., & Kim, J. H. (2014). The relationships among emotional intelligence, interpersonal relationship, and job satisfaction of clinical nurses. *The Journal of Korean Academic Society of Nursing Education, 20*(3), 413–423. https://doi.org/10.5977/jkasne.2014.20.3.413

Lee, Y. B., & Ko, M. S. (2015). The effect of clinical nurses' communication competency and emotional intelligence on organizational performance. *Journal of Korean Clinical Nursing Research, 21*(3), 347–354. https://doi.org/10.22650/JKCNR.2015.21.3.347

Madadkhani, Z., & Nikoogoftar, M. (2015). Critical thinking in nurses: Predictive role of emotional intelligence. *Hayat, 20*(4), 77–88.

Marzuki, N. A., Justaffa, C. S., & Matsaad, Z. (2015). Emotional intelligence: Its relations to communication and information technology skills. *Asian Social Science, 11*(15). https://doi.org/10.5539/ass.v11n15p267

Oh, E. J., Lee, M. H., & Ko, S. H. (2016). Influence of emotional intelligence and empathy on the facilitative communication ability of psychiatric nurses. *Journal of Korean Academy of psychiatric and Mental Health Nursing, 25*(4), 283–293. https://doi.org/10.12934/jkpmhn.2016.25.4.283

Rego, A., Godinho, L., McQueen, A., & Cunha, M. P. (2008). Emotional intelligence and caring behaviour in nursing. *Service Industries Journal, 30*(9), 1419–1437. https://doi.org/10.1080/02642060802621486

Zhu, B., Chen, C.-R., Shi, Z.-Y., Liang, H.-X., & Liu, B. (2016). Mediating effect of self-efficacy in relationship between emotional intelligence and clinical communication competency of nurses. *International Journal of Nursing Sciences, 3*(2), 162–168. https://doi.org/10.1016/j.ijnss.2016.04.003

EI and Stress, Burnout

Farmer, S. (2004). *The relationship of emotional intelligence to burnout and job satisfaction among nurses in early nursing practice.* The University of Utah, ProQuest Dissertations Publishing, 3141849.

Gerits, L., Derksen, J., & Verbruggenm, A. (2004). Emotional intelligence and adaptive success of nurses. *Mental Retardation, 42*(2), 106–121. https://doi.org/10.1352/0047-6765(2004)42<106:EIAASO>2.0.CO;2

Go, N., Park, K. S., & Im, Y. S. (2016). A study on the mediating effect of emotional intelligence between perfectionism and burnout in advanced practice nurses (APN). *Journal of Korean Academy of Nursing Administration, 22*(2), 109–118. https://doi.org/10.11111/jkana.2016.22.2.109

Görgens Ekermans, G., & Brand, T. (2012). Emotional intelligence as a moderator in the stress–burnout relationship: A questionnaire study on nurses. *Journal of Clinical Nursing, 21*(15), 2275–2285. https://doi.org/10.1111/j.1365-2702.2012.04171.x

Huang, H., Liu, L., Yang, S., Cui, X., Zhang, J., & Wu, H. (2019). Effects of job conditions, occupational stress, and emotional intelligence on chronic fatigue among Chinese nurses: A cross-sectional study. *Psychology Research and Behavior Management, 12*, 351–360. https://doi.org/10.2147/prbm.s207283

Landa, J., Lopez Zafra, E., Martos, M., & Aguilar Luzon, M. C. (2008). The relationship between emotional intelligence, occupational stress and health in nurses: A questionnaire survey. *International Journal of Nursing Studies, 45*, 888–901. https://doi.org/10.1016/j.ijnurstu.2007.03.005

Nabirye, R., Brown, K., Pryor, E., & Maples, E. (2011). Occupational stress, job satisfaction and job performance among hospital nurses in Kampala, Uganda. *Journal of Nursing Management, 19*(6), 760–768. https://doi.org/10.1111/J.1365-2834.2011.01240.x

Park, J., & Oh, J. (2019). Influence of perceptions of death, end-of-life care stress, and emotional intelligence on attitudes towards end-of-life care among nurses in the neonatal intensive care unit. *Child Health Nursing Research, 25*(1), 38–47. https://doi.org/10.4094/chnr.2019.25.1.38

Por, J., Barriball, L., Fitzpatrick, J., & Roberts, J. (2011). Emotional intelligence: Its relationship to stress, coping, well-being and professional performance in nursing students. *Nurse Education Today, 31*(8), 855–860. https://doi.org/10.1016/j.nedt.2010.12.023

Shujuan, X., Shenghong, H., Meihong, Z., & Huahua, C. (2019). The role of emotional intelligence in relieving work pressure for practice nurses: A cross-sectional study. *American Journal of Nursing Science, 8*(2), 36–42. https://doi.org/10.11648/j.ajns.20190802.11

EI and Patient Safety, Customer Satisfaction, Quality Care

Cummings, G., Hayduk, L., & Estabrooks, C. (2005). Mitigating the impact of hospital restructuring on nurses: The responsibility of emotionally intelligent leadership. *Nursing Research, 54*(1), 2–12. https://doi.org/10.1097/00006199-200501000-00002

Ranjbar Ezzatabadi, M., Bahrami, M. A., Hadizadeh, F., Arab, M., Nasiri, S., Amiresmaili, M., & Tehrani, A. G. (2012). Nurses' emotional intelligence impact on the quality of hospital services. *Iranian Red Crescent Medical Journal, 14*(12), 758–763. https://doi.org/10.5812/ircmj.926

Willard, S. (2006). Relationship of emotional intelligence and adherence to combination antiretroviral medications by individuals living with HIV disease. *Journal of the Association of Nurses in AIDS Care, 17*(2), 16–26. https://doi.org/10.1016/j.jana.2006.01.001

Yalcin, B., Karahan, T., Ozcelik, M., & Igde, F. (2008). The effects of an emotional intelligence program on the quality of life and well-being of patients with type 2 diabetes mellitus. *The Diabetes Educator, 34*, 1013. https://doi.org/10.1177/0145721708327303

EI and Nursing Students

Ahn, S.-Y., Kim, Y.-J., & Wong, H. J. (2017a). The influence of emotional intelligence and satisfaction in major on mental health among nursing students. *Journal of Advanced Research in Dynamical and Control Systems, 9*(9 Special Issue), 163–169.

Ahn, S.-Y., Kim, Y.-J., & Wong, H.-J. (2017b). The influence of mental health, emotional intelligence, and self-directed learning ability on interpersonal relationships among nursing students. *Journal of Advanced Research in Dynamical and Control Systems, 9*(9 Special Issue), 580–589.

Åž enyuva, E., Kaya, H., IÅŸik, B., & Bodur, G. (2014). Relationship between self-compassion and emotional intelligence in nursing students. *International Journal of Nursing Practice, 20*(6), 588–596. https://doi.org/10.1111/Ijn.12204

Beauvais, A., Brady, N., O'Shea, E. R., & Quin Griffen, M. T. (2011). Emotional intelligence and nursing performance among nursing students. *Nurse Education Today, 31*(4), 396–401. https://doi.org/10.1016/j.nedt.2010.07.013

Fernandez, R., Salamonson, Y., & Griffiths, R. (2012). Emotional intelligence as a predictor of academic performance in first year accelerated graduate entry nursing students. *Journal of Clinical Nursing, 21*(23–24), 3485–3492. https://doi.org/10.1111/j.1365-2702.2012.04199.x

Fitzpatrick, J. J. (2016). Helping nursing students develop and expand their emotional intelligence. *Nursing Education Perspectives, 37*, 124. https://doi.org/10.1097/01.NEP.0000000000000020

John, B., & Al-Sawad, M. (2015). Perceived stress in clinical areas and emotional intelligence among baccalaureate nursing students. *Journal of the Indian Academy of Applied Psychology, 41*(Special Issue 3), 75–84.

Jung, G.-H., Ham, Y.-S., & Lee, D.-Y. (2018). Emotional intelligence and interpersonal relationship according to color preference of Korean nursing students. *Asia Life Sciences, 15*(1), 449–457.

Kim, M. S. (2018). Influence of metacognition and emotional intelligence on self-leadership in nursing students. *Journal of Korean Academy of Nursing Administration, 25*(2), 146. https://doi.org/10.11111/jkana.2019.25.2.146

Lana, A., Baizán, E. M., Faya-Ornia, G., & López, M. L. (2015). Emotional intelligence and health risk behaviors in nursing students. *Journal of Nursing Education, 54*(8), 464–467. https://doi.org/10.3928/01484834-20150717-08

Lee, O. S., & Gu, M. O. (2014). Development and effects of emotional intelligence program for undergraduate nursing students: Mixed methods research. *Journal of Korean Academy of Nursing, 44*(6), 682–696. https://doi.org/10.4040/jkan.2014.44.6.682

Marvos, C., & Hale, F. (2015). Emotional intelligence and clinical performance/retention of nursing students. *Asia Pacific Journal of Oncology Nursing, 2*(2), 63–71. https://doi.org/10.4103/2347-5625.157569

Meng, L., & Qi, J. (2018). The effect of an emotional intelligence intervention on reducing stress and improving communication skills of nursing students. *NeuroQuantology, 16*(1), 37–42. https://doi.org/10.14704/nq.2018.16.1.1175

Rankin, B. (2013). Emotional intelligence: Enhancing values-based practice and compassionate care in nursing. *Journal of Advanced Nursing, 69*(12), 2717–2725. https://doi.org/10.1111/jan.12161

Rice, E. (2015). Predictors of successful clinical performance in associate degree nursing students. *Nurse Educator, 40*(4), 207–211. https://doi.org/10.1097/nne.0000000000000136

Roso-Bas, F., Jimenez, A. P., & Garcia-Buades, E. (2016). Emotional variables, dropout, and academic performance in Spanish nursing students. *Nurse Education Today, 37*, 53–58. https://doi.org/10.1016/j.nedt.2015.11.021

EPILOGUE

As the story goes, Florence Nightingale arrived at the newly built, wooden, single-story field hospital during the Crimean war, accompanied by her cadre of newly minted nurses. The physicians would not let them in. In the care model of the day, only physicians delivered patient care.

Undeterred, Florence and the other nurses set up camp, made their meals, and waited. The wounded came and, still, they were not allowed to enter the hospital. They waited and trained, with the new nurses listening to Florence talk about how to care for the sick. More wounded came. The nurses waited. As that horrible war continued, wounded soldiers poured in until the hospital was overflowing with the sick, dying, and dead. At some point, the physicians, completely overwhelmed, allowed the nurses entry.

The world has never been the same. Like the first patient anesthetized with ether under a skylight at Massachusetts General Hospital, like that first dose of antibiotic administered, or the first vaccine ever used, the axis of the world of healthcare shifted in that moment. It was a pivot point in the history of nursing.

Florence and her nurses administered her odd treatments, like giving the sick and wounded food. Imagine that—giving food, typically saved for fighting soldiers, instead to those likely to die anyway! Outlandish. Florence instituted handwashing, hydration, and clean air and water. Before Florence's arrival, a wounded soldier who arrived at the hospital alive had a 42% chance of dying. When she left, it had dropped to 2%. As much as any moment in history, in that field hospital, nursing became nursing.

In 2020, the COVID-19 pandemic swept across the world. In a short matter of weeks, life changed, and the nursing profession turned on a pivot point again. No one knows how many of the roughly 35 million nurses worldwide cared for those infected. From New York City to Kabul, from the highest tech ICU in Berlin to African villages without electricity or running water, nurses did the best they could with what was available. We will never know how many became sick and infected those they loved as a result. The number who died because they put caring for others above their own safety will also never be known. These pandemic nurses have redefined nursing professionalism. Their experience has pointed out clearly what we must do next. The path is not ambiguous. The only question is, will we do what is required?

Our grief for the nurses who suffered and died is overwhelming. Our rage reading Facebook posts that nurses write after caring for patients without proper protective equipment, and their grief at not being able to do more for those dying alone, is also overwhelming. But our grief and rage are not sufficient. These feelings are not enough to honor our colleagues, alive and dead. We honor them by taking action, by doing justice to this pivot point in the history of nursing.

If not now, when? Once again, we must push open a closed door, step inside, and do that thing we do. We must use the tools we have, pick up ones we never tried, and invent new ones. Emotional intelligence (EI) abilities are examples of such tools. These tools will help us with work that is ahead. The work is this:

1. Conversion of the U.S. healthcare system from a for-profit industry to a public service
2. Healing the trauma of COVID-19 caregivers
3. Advocacy for marginalized populations not served by the current U.S. healthcare system
4. A new kind of ethics of practice that substitutes self-care for self-sacrifice.

EMOTIONAL INTELLIGENCE AND HEALTHCARE REFORM

As this book goes to print, more than 230,000 people in the United States have died of COVID-19. No one knows what will happen next. You roll your eyes because by the time you read this, you will know. Maybe it gets better fast. Maybe the pandemic receded, life returned to normal, and a vaccine was found. Or, maybe things got much, worse than we imagined. Maybe the world pulled together. Maybe it didn't.

Regardless, it is put-up-or-shut-up time for the nursing profession. We can't go back to "normal" because the truth is, normal was not working, as the pandemic made painfully clear. By most objective measures, Italy had one of the best healthcare systems in the world. It was completely overwhelmed anyway. In the United States, in for-profit hospitals, ICU beds were expensive and therefore not sufficient for emergencies, and patients died for lack of ICU equipment, treatments, and care. Uninsured people avoided care when they were sick because of the cost of COVID-19 screening. Elders died in nursing homes that had never been safe. People of color died faster and in greater numbers than others in our country. To deal with the pandemic, we built field hospitals in parks, put

ICU beds in hospital cafeterias. Wearing a mask to protect others became so highly politicized that the virus spread where it should have been easily controlled. One Irish reporter said, "We have loved the United States, and envied her. But now all we feel is pity."

The need for change, and rapid change, is upon us. EI skills will help. Conflict, blame, finger-pointing, xenophobia, and the negative effects of grief are all inevitable. It will consume us, even if things get better right away. Nurses must not let this distract from the work of change at hand. EI will help us do this. EI is not a "soft skill." It is a shovel. It is practical. It will help us do what needs doing. Like shovels in the hands of first responders at the pile on 911, it will help us dig out, deal with the damage, and start to rebuild. To continue to care for our patients, our, friends, families, neighbors, and ourselves, we will need that shovel. It will help us clear away the rubble of the disaster upon us and build the future. Will we do this or not?

EMOTIONAL INTELLIGENCE AND WOUNDED HEALERS

Whatever happens next, there is healing to do. For those of us who can bear to, read Facebook entries written after 12-, 14-, 16-hour shifts under horrific conditions. They are heartbreaking, inspiring, uplifting, emotionally crushing. I read them, wondering, what will happen to this person next? Will they be able to dip into a deep well of resilience and live, whole and well, long after this experience? Will this experience break them, causing lasting trauma and emotional damage? Even if they continue to work, will we have lost them? Is this pandemic a seminal event in nursing that will form a generation of nurse advocates such as the world has never seen, or will they be a burned-out, traumatized lost generation? What are we going to do to help them?

After COVID-19 has done its worst, nurses may leave the profession in droves, and who could blame them? To lose a generation of wisdom, experience, and expertise would be an incalculable catastrophe. The workforce implications of their loss, and the difficulty of recruiting young people who witnessed what this generation faced, may result in a nursing shortage at a time when the continued effects of the virus increase demand for nurses.

Evidence from 25 years of research, from common sense and practical observation, show EI skills can be used for healing. Whether for trauma care, PTSD, or healing by just plainly listening, the skills of identifying emotions, understanding them, using them to reason, and managing them are practical, specific, and useful in healing these wounded healers.

EMOTIONAL INTELLIGENCE AND ADVOCACY

EI Skills are advocacy skills. Protesting ICU nurses in Phoenix, Arizona, and New York City, who after working 12-hour shifts in war zone conditions, identified their anger, understood its power to self-injure or motivate, and used their emotions to reason and manage their emotions. They did not make counter-protest signs to confront protestors who said COVID-19 was a hoax. They did not scream back at those who yelled at them. They put on their masks and scrubs and stood in the street. They stood up for those who could not stand up and were joined by others across the world. If you still aren't sure what EI looks like in practice, look at those pictures. EI skills work in conflict. They are powerful skills for advocacy. We know this from research, from common sense, and from practical observation. Those nurses in Phoenix and New York City likely neither know nor care what EI is, but they should be the poster children for it, the exemplars. Their skills show us a way forward. Inspired by their wisdom and courage, will we use skills like theirs or not?

EMOTIONAL INTELLIGENCE AND THE ETHICS OF SELF-CARE

Nurses assigned COVID-19 patients on ventilators, patients who were at very high risk for contagion, were given PPE equipment that would not protect them. They refused to enter the ICU and were promptly suspended. Let us be clear. There was a formal disciplinary procedure that threatened their jobs because they refused to comply with a well-known threat to their lives, and the lives of their loved ones. Do nurses have the legal, ethical, and moral right to protect their own lives? Not on that day. Not in that hospital. In the heat of the epidemic, when they had plenty to do, nurse protestors stood before the U.S. Capitol holding over their heads the pictures of nurses who had died of coronavirus. Our grief at the sight of this is not enough. Our grief is not sufficient to the time. We owe those nurses and future nurses a change in ethical standards for professional practice. To risk the life of a nurse should be considered unethical, and to defend ones' own health should be considered not just acceptable, but required. The ANA Code of Ethics demands this, but when will this demand become standard practice?

How do we do all these things? How do we support the healing of those whose caring for pandemic victims wounded them? How do we begin the insistent work of reforming healthcare in the United States? How do we transform the ethical standards of our profession so that dedication to caring does not necessitate personal risk?

The message in the research is clear, so what will we do? The body of nursing EI research is by no means comprehensive. There is considerable work to be done. Yet, it is built on a solid foundation of research from other disciplines and the whole body of it together: EI makes a difference. These abilities, which are clear, measurable, and can be both learned and improved, make us better, safer, and more effective nurses. Will we use them or not?

INDEX

Printed in the United States
by Baker & Taylor Publisher Services